THE TRANS FAT REMEDY

*The First Consumer Guide to Your
Family's Biggest Health Threat*

THE TRANS FAT REMEDY

The First Consumer Guide to Your Family's Biggest Health Threat

Deborah Mitchell

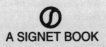

A SIGNET BOOK

SIGNET
Published by New American Library, a division of
Penguin Group (USA) Inc., 375 Hudson Street,
New York, New York 10014, U.S.A.
Penguin Books Ltd, 80 Strand,
London WC2R 0RL, England
Penguin Books Australia Ltd, 250 Camberwell Road,
Camberwell, Victoria 3124, Australia
Penguin Books Canada Ltd, 10 Alcorn Avenue,
Toronto, Ontario, Canada M4V 3B2
Penguin Books (NZ), cnr Airborne and Rosedale Roads,
Albany, Auckland 1310, New Zealand

Penguin Books Ltd, Registered Offices:
80 Strand, London WC2R 0RL, England

First published by Signet, an imprint of New American Library,
a division of Penguin Group (USA) Inc.

First Printing, August 2004
10 9 8 7 6 5 4 3 2 1

PUBLISHER'S NOTES
Every effort as been made to ensure that the information contained in this book is complete and accurate. However, neither the publisher nor the author is engaged in rendering
professional advice or services to the individual reader. The ideas, procedures, and sugges-
tions contained in this book are not intended as a substitute for consulting with your
physician. All matters regarding your health require medical supervision. Neither the author nor the publisher shall be liable or responsible for any loss or damage allegedly
arising from any information or suggestion in this book.

The recipes contained in this book are to be followed exactly as written. The publisher is
not responsible for your specific health or allergy needs that may require medical supervision. The publisher is not responsible for any adverse reactions to the recipes contained
in this book.

While the author has made every effort to provide accurate telephone numbers and Internet addresses at the time of publication, neither the publisher nor the author assumes
any responsibility for errors, or for changes that occur after publication.

For
Pumpernickle, Shiloh, Jazz, Rama,
Buddha, Boomer, Gypsy, Toby,
Sasha, and The Bear

Contents

CHAPTER 1

What You Need to Know to Avoid Franken Fats

Just when you thought you had "the fat dilemma" figured out—that saturated fats are bad, polyunsaturated and monounsaturated fats are good, and you should keep your total daily fat intake to less than 30 percent—*now* you're being told you have to avoid trans fats because they are likely even *more* dangerous to your health than are saturated fats.

Where did these trans fats come from? Are they something new? Why didn't anyone warn us about them before now? How can you identify trans fats in the foods you eat? How dangerous are they? And most important, what foods should you buy and which ones should you avoid—at the supermarket and when eating out—to help keep you and your family healthy?

This book answers all of these questions and more. First, we show you how to read and decipher the nutritional and ingredient information on your food packages to determine the amounts of trans fats and other fats in the items. The Food and Drug Administration (FDA) has required all food manufacturers to list the amount of trans fats on their packaging by January 1, 2006. Until then, you will have to play "detective" in many cases to discern the amount of trans fats in the items you buy. Don't worry: We'll show you how to do that.

Then, this book does what no other book does: It takes you on a virtual trip through the supermarket, aisle by aisle, and identifies foods that contain significant amounts of trans fats, as well as those that contain none or a minute amount (less than 0.5 gram per serving). Say you want to buy peanut butter; which brands are high in trans fats and which ones are healthy? Are there any healthy crunchy snacks you can buy for your family? Which cookies are lowest in bad fats? Are the breakfast bars you've been buying for your family the healthiest choice you can make? Which salad dressings are the wisest choice for your family? Are any of those frozen breakfast or dinner meals really healthy? You can literally take this book with you to the market and use it as a guide as you go up and down the aisles.

Finally, because you, like most Americans, probably eat out fairly often, this book takes you on a virtual restaurant tour and helps you identify which foods are your healthiest and safest bets when eating away from home—and away from ingredient labels and Nutrition Facts panels you can check to see fat levels and other nutritional information.

This book is important for people of all ages, but if you have children, it is especially critical. Why? Because children are the biggest consumers of foods that are highest in trans fats—foods such as cookies, snack cakes, candy, crackers, peanut butter, pizza, processed breakfast cereals, french fries, potato chips, and corn chips. This book can help you choose healthier options for your children and assist in establishing good dietary habits that can last a lifetime.

WHAT ARE TRANS FATS?

You may be familiar with the term "franken foods," coined during the 1990s to describe foods that are genetically modified and thus, to some extent, unnatural. But decades before franken foods entered the marketplace, "franken fats" were becoming part of your food. These franken fats, or trans fats, are a synthetic byproduct of a chemical process called "hydrogenation." Hydrogenation produces fats that have an abnormal, and unnatural, molecular structure that is foreign to the body and, as you'll read below, introduces many health concerns. However, hydrogenation is popular among food manufacturers because it saves them money.

Thus it's no surprise that trans fats are found in some of the most popular foods consumed in the United States, including baked goods (cookies, cakes, pies, breads, rolls), margarines, crackers, potato chips, french fries, peanut butter, breakfast bars, packaged dinners, soups, and especially fast food. In the following chapters you'll learn more about trans fats and, most important, how to avoid them and choose healthier alternatives, like whole foods, minimally processed foods, or easy, nutritious recipes you can make at home. **Note:** Trans fats are also found naturally in animal foods—meat, poultry, and dairy products—but generally in lesser amounts than seen in foods that contain hydrogenated oils. Since animal foods also contain saturated fats, they present a double health hazard. We discuss naturally occurring trans fats in chapter 2. First, however, let's find out how trans fats are made.

HYDROGENATION

Hydrogenation is a chemical method that was originally developed in the 1900s as a way to produce low-cost soap. But researchers quickly found other uses for the process, and by around 1905, hydrogenation was being used by the food industry to transform liquid vegetable oils into hydrogenated fats, resulting in hard margarine.

Trans fats are formed during hydrogenation, a process that takes relatively healthy unsaturated vegetable oil and turns it into a health-damaging solid. To accomplish this, hydrogen atoms are forced into the molecules of unsaturated vegetable oils using tremendous pressure, high heat (about 250 to 400 degrees Fahrenheit) for several hours, and a metal catalyst (usually nickel), which allow the hydrogen atoms to "stick" to the unsaturated oil molecules. The process of adding hydrogen atoms to unsaturated fats causes the formation of dozens of new, unnatural compounds, including trans fats.

Hydrogenated Oil vs. Partially Hydrogenated Oil

To make best use of hydrogenation, food manufacturers only partially hydrogenate vegetable oils. That is, they add only enough hydrogen atoms to reach the consistency they need for their products. That's why in most cases you'll see "partially hydrogenated vegetable oil" or "partially hydrogenated vegetable shortening" on food labels instead of "hydrogenated oil or fat." Generally, hydrogenated oil or fat is too hard for use in most food products, although you will see it in some items, such as some peanut butters and baked goods.

HYDROGENATION: PROS AND CONS

For almost a century, many people viewed hydrogenation as a good thing. Certainly food manufacturers did. Now, however, has come the time to weigh the pros and cons of hydrogenation in light of its byproduct—trans fats.

Benefits of Hydrogenation

The benefits of hydrogenation in the food industry come down to one word—economics. Food manufacturers like hydrogenated fats because:

- They are cheaper to use than butter or coconut oil, and have been more accepted by consumers than other possible replacements, including lard and beef fat.
- Hydrogenation increases the amount of time it takes before oils become rancid, which means foods that contain hydrogenated oils—and thus trans fats—have a longer shelf life. Items that can stay on the shelves longer mean better profits for manufacturers. This is a major consideration for manufacturers who ship their products overseas and for stores and warehouses that like to stockpile products, a very common practice in the United States.
- Hydrogenation improves texture and "creaminess" of foods. Thus foods that contain hydrogenated fats feel good in your mouth.

Hydrogenated vegetable oil proved to be a boon to restaurants. At one time, restaurants used beef fat in their deep commercial fryers. This saturated animal fat quickly turned to liquid in the 350 degrees or higher in the fryers. When use of beef fat—which is very high in unhealthy saturated fat—became unpopular because of its association with heart disease and obesity, vegetable oil became the option. However, vegetable oil has a high content of unsaturated fat, and when it breaks down in the fryer, it produces toxic substances that can change the taste and color of food. These were obviously not desirable effects, so restaurant owners found a new answer—hydrogenated oil. Hydrogenated vegetable oil resists breakdown in the high temperatures of deep-fat fryers, which allows restaurants to reuse the oil for a month or more before they change it—an obvious financial savings.

If hydrogenation could do all these things and not produce harmful byproducts or adverse health effects, then there would be no need for this book or for the Food and Drug Administration to require labeling of trans fats. But the reality is, hydrogenation has a number of serious downsides.

Health Hazards of Hydrogenation and Trans Fats

Perhaps the most significant danger associated with hydrogenation is that the trans fats it produces are linked with an increased risk of heart disease, the number one killer of men and women in the United States. Approximately 42.2 million Americans have heart disease, and another 1.1 million experience a heart attack or other heart-related event every year. Of those 1.1 million, nearly 50 percent of them will die. In addition to causing the death of more than 500,000 Americans per year, heart disease also takes a huge financial toll. In 2002, heart disease cost $214 billion, including $115 billion in direct medical costs, according to Tommy G. Thompson, Secretary of Health and Human Services.

We talk more in depth about how trans fats increase your risk of heart disease in chapter 2, where we compare trans fats with saturated fats. For now, you should know that some other downsides to trans fats include:

- They increase insulin resistance, which increases people's tendency to develop type II diabetes. An estimated 17 million Americans have type II diabetes, and the vast majority of them are overweight.
- They have been linked with breast cancer.
- They interfere with the normal function of certain fatty acids, which are essential for health.
- They reduce the quality of breast milk.
- They interfere with pregnancy.
- They reduce the efficiency of the immune system.
- They decrease testosterone levels (only shown in animals thus far).

One problem with trans fats is that they are unnatural, and so the body doesn't deal with them as it does natural substances. This means trans fats stay in the body for a long time and can cause digestive problems and weight gain. Another problem is that these fats break down into prostaglandins, chemicals that cause inflammation. Thus trans fats can also contribute to pain and chronic inflammatory conditions, such as arthritis and, as we've mentioned, heart disease, which is now recognized as a disease that involves inflammation of the blood vessels.

If you have children, you should know that trans fats are especially harmful for young people. Kids love the foods that have the highest levels of trans fats—

foods like french fries, breakfast bars, cookies, crackers, peanut butter, doughnuts, potato chips, candy, and cereals. Although it is true that, in terms of percentage, growing children need more fat than adults, the majority of that fat should be *healthy* fat—preferably monounsaturated fats, less so polyunsaturated fats, and certainly not trans fats and saturated fats. Many experts believe that the growing problems of obesity in children and increasing numbers of children who have high blood pressure, type II diabetes, and heart problems—and some say even attention deficit hyperactivity disorder and other behavioral problems—are associated with high amounts of unhealthy fat in the diet.

BOTTOM LINE

Hydrogenation is a process that produces trans fats, which don't have any redeeming value when it comes to your health. Trans fats are unnatural and unhealthy, and you need to eliminate them as much as possible from your diet and that of your children. In the next chapter, we'll talk more about trans fats and their health effects, as well as how they relate with the other three members of the fat family: saturated, polyunsaturated, and monounsaturated fats.

CHAPTER 2

Comparing Bad Fats and Good Fats

By now you know that trans fats are bad, and in this chapter we're going to tell you just *how* bad they are when it comes to your health. While we're at it, we're going to compare trans fats with the other "bad fat boy"—saturated fats—and explain how they are similar to and different from trans fats. When you are through with this chapter, you will know all you need to know about these two bad fats. You will also be ready to learn how to read nutrition and ingredient labels on the foods you buy for yourself and your family, which we discuss in detail in chapter 3.

But wait; not all fats are bad. Gone are the days when we lumped all fats into one scary category and declared them off-limits. Some fats, namely monounsaturated (like those in olives, olive oil, and flaxseed oil) and, to a lesser extent, polyunsaturated (like those found in some fish), are beneficial when consumed in moderation, and in fact are necessary for good health. You need to learn about these fats as well, as you will see them on some food labels. Therefore this chapter concludes with a discussion of polyunsaturated and monounsaturated fats and how to include them—instead of trans fats and saturated fats—in your diet.

WHAT IS FAT?

Fats are composed of long chains of carbon atoms that are attached to each other with either single or double arms (or bonds) and to hydrogen with single bonds. The number of hydrogen molecules that attach themselves to the carbon arms, and where they attach, determine whether the fat is saturated, polyunsaturated, or monounsaturated. All three of these fats occur naturally and have standardized structures. Trans fats, however, are artificially produced, and their structure is unnatural and thus alien to the body and a health risk.

It's important to remember that *all* foods (except refined sugar) contain at least a miniscule amount of fat, even a carrot or stalk of celery, and that all types of fat appear together in every food item. One type of fat, however, usually dominates. Thus butter, which is 66 percent saturated fat, 4 percent polyunsaturated fat, and 30 percent monounsaturated fat, is primarily composed of saturated fat, while olive oil is only 14 percent saturated fat but contains 77 percent monounsaturated and 9 percent polyunsaturated fats. Foods such as kidney beans, carrots, peaches, and lentils, and hundreds of other fruits, vegetables, grains, and legumes, however, are considered to be fat free, because they contain only miniscule amounts of fat.

WHAT'S THE DIFFERENCE BETWEEN FAT AND OIL?

Fat and oil are both types of *lipids*. The only thing that separates a fat from an oil is temperature. That means, a fat (such as margarine, butter, shortening, lard) is solid at room temperature, while an oil is liquid at room temperature.

WHY YOU NEED FAT

Despite the negative response most people have when they hear the word "fat," it's important that you think of it like any other nutrient, like carbohydrates, protein, vitamins, and minerals: It has its good and bad points. If you consume too much protein or vitamin A, or the wrong kind of protein or mineral, for example, it can have negative effects on your health just as can eating the wrong kind of fat. However, good sources of protein or fat, as well as recommended levels of vitamins or minerals, can provide many health benefits.

That being said, let's look at the benefits you get from including good fats in your diet:

- Fats are a major energy source for the body.
- They help the body absorb vitamins A, D, E, and K, and carotenoids.
- The production of critical hormones called "eicosanoids" requires fats.
- Fats aid in proper growth and development.

- For children up to the age of two years—the age group that has the greatest energy needs per unit of body weight than any other age group—fats are a critical source of calories and nutrients.
- Fats are essential for proper brain function; the brain is composed of 17 percent fat. Fat insulates the electrical pathways in the brain and thus ensures its efficient functioning.

The caveat with fats is that you need to consume moderate amounts of good fat and much smaller amounts of bad fat. We talk about how much fat is healthy in the next chapter, but for now, let's discuss the four different types of fats—two good and two bad.

BAD FATS: TRANS AND SATURATED FATS

You already know that trans fats begin as an unsaturated fat, which is transformed into a franken fat by bombarding it with hydrogen atoms to make it partially saturated (hence the words "partially hydrogenated vegetable oil/shortening" you see on food labels) and solid. It's that very unnatural process that makes trans fats so harmful to the body. In particular, trans fats have been linked with a greater risk of heart disease.

How do they do this? Researchers have found that trans fats:

- increase your level of bad cholesterol (low-density lipoprotein, or LDL). This is the type of cholesterol that causes atherosclerosis (hardening of the arteries) and heart disease.

- decrease your level of good cholesterol (high-density lipoprotein, or HDL). You need adequate levels of HDL because this kind of cholesterol helps remove LDL from blood vessels.
- increase your level of triglycerides. Triglycerides are a type of fat that is produced in the liver and is also obtained through your diet. The higher your triglyceride level, the greater tendency your blood has to clot, and your body's natural clot-clearing process is also compromised.
- increase levels of C-reactive protein, a substance that causes inflammation of the blood vessels and thus is a significant factor in heart disease.
- have a detrimental effect on metabolic processes in the heart, which can contribute to heart disease.

Researchers base these findings on the results of various studies. Perhaps most influential is a study that followed more than 85,000 women. In this study, investigators found that there was significantly higher intake of trans-fatty acids among those women who developed heart disease. And in a report put out by the Harvard Medical School, it is estimated that *each year* in the United States, 30,000 to 100,000 premature deaths due to coronary heart disease can be attributed to trans fats and hydrogenation.

Other Health Hazards of Trans Fats

In chapter 1, we briefly mentioned some of the other health concerns associated with trans fats. One we did not mention is the fact that trans fats cause the liver to produce thickened bile. Bile is essential for the efficient digestion of fat. When bile becomes abnormally thick, however, it causes congestion in the gallbladder, which can result in the formation of gallstones, which may need to be removed surgically. Gallbladder congestion also disrupts digestion, which can lead to weight gain.

Several studies also suggest that consumption of trans fats increases the risk of developing cancer. The reason may be the ability of these unnatural fats to disrupt the natural cell membranes and allow cancer-causing elements to invade cells and damage the nucleus. Evidence also suggests that trans fats increase cancer risk by affecting the immune system and hormone balance in the body. Specifically, high consumption of trans fats has been associated with an increased risk of colon cancer, and a Dutch study found a higher concentration of trans fats in the breasts of women who had breast cancer.

If you're pregnant or breastfeeding, trans fats can be a problem as well. Research shows that pregnant women who had high levels of trans fats had *seven times* the risk of preeclampsia (a complication of pregnancy characterized by high blood pressure and edema). If you eat a lot of trans fats and you're breastfeeding, you may be passing those fats to your infant, and there's evidence that infants who are exposed to trans fats through breast milk have impaired brain development and visual acuity.

Saturated Fats

Saturated fats are the ones that give fat a bad name, probably because saturated fats are associated with clogged arteries and heart attacks. Like trans fats, saturated fats raise your level of LDL cholesterol. They also promote increased blood clotting, which in turn contributes to strokes, heart attack, and blood clots in the legs and lungs. The health hazards of saturated fats have been recognized for many years, which is one reason why the Food and Drug Administration required that the amount of saturated fat be listed on Nutrition Facts panels.

But even saturated fats have a good side: Small amounts are necessary because they help the body resist disease and keep cells healthy. Therefore, although it's important to limit your intake of saturated fats—you'll read more about that in the next chapter—you don't want to eliminate them from your diet completely.

Saturated fats are naturally solid at room temperature. They are found primarily in animal products, such as beef, pork, butter, cheese, cream, and poultry, and in some oils derived from plants, including palm oil, coconut oil, vegetable shortening, margarine, and cocoa butter.

THE BETTER FATS: POLYUNSATURATED AND MONOUNSATURATED FATS

Polyunsaturated and monounsaturated fats are commonly placed into the category of "good fats," and compared with trans and saturated fats, they are. However, the label "good fats" can be misleading, as some people may think they can eat as much of these fats as they wish. Even though polyunsaturated and monounsaturated fats are *better* than the bad fats, moderation is the critical thing to remember. We talk more about how much of each type of fat is healthy to eat in chapter 3. For now, let's look at what's good about these better fats.

Polyunsaturated Fats

Polyunsaturated fats are somewhere in between the bad fats and the best fats—monounsaturated. That's because even though polyunsaturated fats are low in saturated fat, they are unstable because of how their carbon and hydrogen bonds are structured. Their instability makes them susceptible to oxidation, which produces free radicals—molecules that can cause cell damage.

Fortunately, there are two classes of polyunsaturated fats—omega-3 fatty acids and omega-6 fatty acids—and one of them is healthy. Without getting into the complicated chemistry of these two types of fatty acids, let's just say that omega-6 fatty acids are generally unhealthy while omega-3 fatty acids are beneficial. Not surprisingly, Americans eat a lot more omega-6 fatty acids than omega-3. You'll find omega-6 fatty acids in meat, as well as in safflower, sunflower, and corn oils. Health risks associated with omega-6 fatty acids include suppression of the immune system, increased incidence of tumors, and inflammation.

Omega-3 fatty acids are believed to help protect you against arthritis, heart disease, hypertension, cancer, diabetes, and stroke. They are found in flaxseed, pumpkin seeds, walnut oil, hempseed oil, some fish—including coldwater fish such as mackerel, tuna, herring, and salmon—and fish oils.

Monounsaturated Fats

Monounsaturated fats are the fats that are usually associated with the Mediterranean diet, in which people typically use a lot of olive oil. In fact, aside from hempseed oil (which is not readily available in some places), olive oil contains a higher amount of monounsaturated fat than any of the oils (see chart). In addition to olive oil, canola oil, peanut oil, and avocado oil also contain a significant amount of monounsaturated fat.

Monounsaturated fats are usually liquid at room temperature, but they may become solid if you refrigerate them. If you keep your olive oil in the refrigerator, you're familiar with this. They are considered to be the more beneficial of the two good fats because they lower LDL and may raise HDL. Research suggests that long-term use of olive oil (which is characteristic of southern Europe) is associated with a low incidence of heart disease.

How to Introduce Good Fats into Your Diet

- Dip your bread in olive oil instead of butter.
- For salad dressing, use olive, flaxseed, canola, or walnut oil. Your healthiest choice is to purchase cold-pressed and unrefined oils.

- Bring your own healthy salad dressings with you when you eat out. You'll find some recipes in chapter 6.

**Breakdown of Fats in Different Oils
(percentages may vary slightly depending on the brand of oil purchased)**

Type of Oil/Fat	Saturated	Polyunsaturated	Monounsaturated
Canola oil	6%	34%	60%
Hempseed oil	8%	12%	80%
Pumpkin seed oil	9%	34%	57%
Flaxseed oil	9%	19%	72%
Safflower oil	10%	77%	13%
Sunflower oil	11%	69%	20%
Corn oil	13%	62%	25%
Olive oil	14%	9%	77%
Soybean oil	15%	61%	24%
Margarine	17%	34%	49%
Peanut oil	18%	33%	49%
Palm oil	52%	11%	37%
Coconut oil	92%	2%	6%
Beef fat	52%	4%	44%
Butter	66%	4%	30%

BOTTOM LINE

Fats are a critical part of your diet because they are necessary for good health. The key to getting the healthy benefits from them is to choose the healthy fats over the unhealthy ones as much as possible, and to be moderate in your intake of the healthy ones as well. Can we define "moderate"? How much of each of the four types of fat should you include in your diet? We answer these and more questions in the next chapter.

CHAPTER 3

How Much Is Too Much and How to Identify Trans Fats

By now you should be convinced that trans fats—and the many processed foods that they are in—are not your friend. You're ready to say "no" to trans fats; you're ready to banish them from your grocery cart and your kitchen and to replace them with healthier, whole foods, which have virtually no trans fats.

But you realize you have two pressing questions. One, how do you know how much trans fats is considered to be healthy and safe to eat? And two, even if you did know the answer to question one, how can you find out how much trans fats are in your food (given that most foods are not yet labeled) so you'll know which foods to avoid?

In this chapter we answer both these questions, so you can feel confident about shopping for yourself and your family. First, however, let's begin with a brief explanation of the ruling made by the Food and Drug Administration—the ruling that has sent food manufacturers scrambling to update their packaging and consumers wondering what it means to them.

THE FDA RULING

On July 9, 2003, the Food and Drug Administration (FDA) published its final ruling that requires manufacturers to list the amount of trans fats on the Nutrition Facts panels of conventional foods and some dietary supplements. Here are the main points of that ruling that will come in handy when it's time for you to shop:

- Manufacturers have until January 1, 2006, to comply with this ruling.
- Manufacturers of conventional foods and some dietary supplements (e.g., energy and nutrition bars) must list the amount of trans fats in their products on a separate line, immediately under the line that gives the amount of saturated fat on the Nutrition Facts panel.
- The amount of trans fats does not have to be listed if the total amount of fat in the food item is less than 0.5 gram per serving, and no claims are made about fat, fatty acids, or cholesterol. If the amount of trans fats is not listed, the manufacturer must give a footnote that states the food is "not a significant source of trans fat."
- Researchers have confirmed that there is a relationship between the amount of trans fats people consume and an increased risk of coronary heart disease. The FDA used information gathered from scientific reports, studies, and expert panels from the National Cholesterol Education Program, the National Institutes of Health, the Insti-

tute of Medicine, and the United States Department of Agriculture. However, they have not identified a Daily Reference Value for trans fats, and so consumers will not be guided as to what the recommended percent Daily Value of trans fats should be in their diet.

- The FDA estimates that by January 1, 2009, this ruling will have prevented from 600 to 1,200 cases of coronary heart disease and 250 to 500 deaths per year. The FDA also believes that if consumers heed the warnings it has issued about trans fats, the new ruling "will save between $900 million and 1.8 billion each year in medical costs, lost productivity, and pain and suffering," as quoted in a July 9, 2003 news release by the U.S. Department of Health and Human Services.

The purpose of the FDA ruling is to help you choose foods that will allow you to keep your intake of trans fats, as well as saturated fats and cholesterol (which are already listed on Nutrition Facts panels), as low as possible. Thus you will be making heart-healthy food choices that will lower your risk of heart disease. It is *not* an effort to make you completely eliminate trans fats from your diet. Total elimination of trans fats from your diet is impractical and unhealthy; even if you were to eliminate foods that contain a significant amount of trans fats, there are still many items that contain minute amounts. Avoiding all of these foods would leave you with a very limited diet, which would likely be unhealthy and unbalanced. Remember: If you follow the recommended intake of 7 to 10 percent (of your total daily calorie intake) of combined saturated and trans fats—which is easy to do if you focus on whole foods and minimally processed foods—you'll be on the right track.

HOW MUCH IS TOO MUCH TRANS FAT?

When the Food and Drug Administration decided to require food manufacturers to list the amount of trans fats on their packaging, it didn't take the next, seemingly logical step: It did not require anyone to make a determination as to how much trans fats people should, or should not, consume.

The agency that has the task of determining what the recommended nutritional levels should be in the U.S. diet is the National Academy of Sciences. However, the academy said that there was not enough scientific information available for them to name a recommended daily intake level for trans fats at this time.

Before the FDA's final ruling was made in July 2003, many advocates of the labeling change had hoped that the FDA would at least require a footnote on packaging that recommended people eat only a little trans fats. Such a footnote will not appear on food labels, however. According to the Grocery Manufacturers of America—a group that lobbied against including the statement on labels—consumer testing indicated that such a statement scared people back to eating foods that are high in saturated fat.

How to Determine a Safe Trans Fat Level for You

"Trans fats are bad fats. The less trans fat you and I eat, the healthier we will be." The sentiment of this statement, made by Secretary of Health and Human Services Tommy G. Thompson during a news conference on July 9, 2003, has been echoed by many experts, including the National Academy of Sciences, the National Heart, Lung, and Blood Institute, and the American Heart Association. Given that research has linked trans fats with an increased risk of heart disease, few people will be surprised by these words.

But how much is "less"? If you're eating 20 grams a day now, is 18 grams okay? After all, 18 *is* less than 20. But we need to back up a moment; you don't even *know* how much trans fats you're eating, because the vast majority of foods are not labeled. What are you supposed to do?

First, let's get some help from the American Heart Association, which has made the following recommendations:

- Saturated fat *plus* trans fat intake should not exceed 10 percent of total caloric intake for healthy people (e.g., people who are not obese or who don't have high cholesterol, high blood pressure, heart disease, diabetes).
- Saturated fat should make up less than 7 percent of total calories for people who have coronary heart disease, high LDL cholesterol (low-density lipoprotein—"bad" cholesterol), or diabetes.

- Your total daily fat intake—including saturated, trans, monounsaturated, and polyunsaturated fats—should be 30 percent or less of total daily calories. **Note:** Some experts recommend total fat intake be closer to 20 percent of total daily calories.

If we consider the information in the first two bullets, we can safely conclude that your intake of trans fats should not exceed 3 percent of your total calories per day.

We can now use these recommendations to make a determination of how much trans fats is considered "healthy" for you. (You will learn how to read and decipher package labels later in this chapter.) To arrive at that number, you first need to know approximately how many calories a day you consume. If you don't know, keep a record in a notebook of everything you consume—meals, snacks, beverages—for two to three days. You can get calorie counts from the packages of items you eat, as well as from books that give calorie counts for packaged, fresh, and fast foods (see Appendix). Once you have counted up your caloric intake for each day, you can use the following chart to identify one, how many total fat grams you should be eating daily, and two, how much of that fat should be saturated *and* trans fats added together (7 to 10 percent total, depending on your health).

THE TRANS FAT REMEDY

Calories Consumed/Day	No. Fat Grams/Day (20–30% of Daily Calories)	No. Sat. + Trans Fat Grams/Day (7–10% of Daily Calories)
1,200	24–36	8–12
1,400	28–42	10–14
1,600	32–48	11–16
1,800	36–54	13–18
2,000	40–60	14–20
2,200	44–66	15–22
2,400	48–72	17–24
2,600	52–78	18–26
2,800	56–84	19–28
3,000	60–90	21–30

Let's say you're a thirty-year-old woman who consumes, on average, 1,600 calories a day. You're always watching your weight, so you decide to limit your total fat consumption to 32 grams (20 percent of calories) per day. You're in good health, so your combined daily intake of saturated and trans fats should not exceed 16 grams, which leaves up to 16 grams of polyunsaturated and monounsaturated fat that you can eat per day.

If you stop at McDonald's on your way to work and pick up a Bacon, Egg & Cheese Biscuit for breakfast, you've just consumed 31 grams of total fat, of which 10 are saturated. That means you've just eaten your entire quota of fat (minus 1 gram) at one meal. If you look at the remaining 21 grams (31 total minus 10 saturated fat equals 21 grams), they consist of trans, polyunsaturated, and monounsaturated fats, each in unknown amounts.

Given that this sandwich is cooked in partially hydrogenated oil and that the biscuit contains partially hydrogenated oil, chances are much, if not most, of the remaining 21 grams are trans fats. (We talk about how to decipher restaurant foods for trans fat content in chapter 4.) That means you have probably just exceeded your total recommended intake of trans fats and saturated fats for the day in one sandwich.

If you decide to pop into a Dunkin' Donuts instead and grab a whole wheat glazed doughnut (whole wheat *must* mean it's healthy, right?), you'll fare somewhat better: only 11 grams of fat, most of which is saturated and trans fats. Although the doughnut seems to be a better choice, you've still consumed nearly all your saturated and trans fat quota for the day (11 out of 16 grams), and it's only breakfast! Clearly, you need some help choosing low trans fat and saturated fat foods. Don't worry: We help you with that task in chapters 4, 5, and 6.

Americans and Trans Fats

How much trans fats do Americans eat every day? The Food and Drug Administration estimates that the average daily intake of trans fats among Americans aged twenty years and older is 5.8 grams, or 2.6 percent, of their total caloric intake per day, which is close to the 3 percent maximum we established. However, other experts place intake closer to nearly four times that amount—approximately 24 grams, or 10 percent of total daily calories. Given our love affair with fast food, margarine, and commercially prepared cakes, cookies, pies, and other baked goods, 24 grams, and even higher, is likely closer to the truth. In fact, according to the FDA, Americans are getting their trans fats from the following sources: 40 percent from baked goods (cookies, breads, crackers, and so on); 21 percent from animal products (meat, poultry, and dairy products all contain trans fats naturally); 17 percent from margarine; 8 percent from fried potatoes; 5 percent from chips and similar snack foods; 4 percent from household shortening; 3 percent from salad dressings; and 1 percent each from breakfast cereals and candy.

What's the best way to minimize your intake of trans fats? Make whole foods—whole grains, beans, legumes, vegetables, fruits, nuts—the mainstay of your diet, and use processed foods, like those that contain trans fats and saturated fats, only occasionally.

Naturally, every person is different and has different dietary habits, so the amount of dietary adjustments each individual makes will vary. What's important now is to determine the amount of trans fats *you're* consuming daily. The rest of this chapter will tell you how to figure out the trans fat content of your food.

HOW TO DECIPHER FOOD LABELS

Until January 1, 2006, when all conventional foods will be required to carry information about its trans fat content, you may have to do some minor detective work to identify the amount of trans fats in the foods you eat. Don't worry: It isn't hard to do, and we're going to show you how.

First, however, let's look at a Nutrition Facts panel. Prior to the FDA ruling on labeling trans fats, food manufacturers were required by the FDA to provide information on the following items: total calories, calories from fat, total fat, saturated fat, cholesterol, sodium, total carbohydrates, dietary fiber, sugars, protein, vitamin A, vitamin C, calcium, and iron. Any other information manufacturers choose to include is optional. Soon, trans fats will be added to the required list.

Note: Labels on foods that are specifically for children younger than two years of age are not required to carry information about saturated fat, polyunsaturated fat, monounsaturated fat, cholesterol, calories from fat, or calories from saturated fat. Labels for infant formulas have their own set of regulations. For an in-depth explanation of the Nutrition Facts panel, see www.cfsan.fda.gov/~dms/fdnewlab.html#nutri.

You can use the information on the Nutrition Facts panel and the ingredient list to figure out, with a good degree of accuracy, how much trans fats a food item contains. Here are some examples of food label information and how to decipher it.

SAMPLES OF FOOD LABEL INFORMATION

The ease with which you can determine the amount of trans fats in any given food item will depend on the food and how much information the manufacturer provides beyond the required levels of total fat and saturated fat. Let's look at several different types of labels you may see in the supermarket.

Sample 1

- Total fat: 5.0 grams
- Saturated fat: 2.0 grams
- Polyunsaturated fat: 1.0 gram
- Monounsaturated fat: 1.5 grams

Because this manufacturer has elected to include information on polyunsaturated and monounsaturated fats along with the required saturated fat information, you may have a good clue as to the amount of trans fats in this item. The three fats listed add up to 4.5 grams, which means there is 0.5 gram "missing." If you see "partially hydrogenated vegetable oil" or "shortening" on the ingredient list, the 0.5 gram may be trans fat. It may, however, be something else, which I explain in the "But It Doesn't Add Up" label.

Sample 2: The "But It Doesn't Add Up" Label

Here is another example of a label where the numbers don't add up to the total fat grams. This happens more often than you think. In this case, the product is Mazola Canola Oil:

- Total fat: 14 grams
- Saturated fat: 1 gram

- Polyunsaturated fat: 4 grams
- Monounsaturated fat: 8 grams

Add it up: $1 + 4 + 8 = 13$. Where's the missing gram? It's in there, but according to FDA regulations, food manufacturers are supposed to *round down* gram figures. In other words, the saturated fat in this product could *actually be* 1.4 grams, polyunsaturated could *actually be* 4.3 grams, and monounsaturated could *actually be* 8.3 grams $(0.4 + 0.3 + 0.3 = 1.0$, the "missing" gram), but the manufacturers rounded down each figure to $1 + 4 + 8$. It's all perfectly legal, but that doesn't mean it isn't confusing. A label like this one could also mean that one or more of the figures has been rounded down but that some of the missing fat is trans fats.

Sample 3: When Zero Doesn't Really Mean Zero

Here's an example of what appears to be deceptive advertising. You will see products, especially margarine-like spreads, that say "0 grams trans fat" on the label, but is that the whole truth? Let's look at a sample label:

- Total fat: 5 grams
- Saturated fat: 1 gram
- Polyunsaturated fat: 2.5 grams
- Monounsaturated fat: 1 gram

When you add up the fats, you get a total of 4.5 grams, not 5 grams. Again, we're looking for the missing

0.5 gram of fat. You may think, "It must be trans fat," yet the label says the product contains "0 grams trans fat."

But then you read the ingredient list, and you see "partially hydrogenated oil" listed. How can that be? The truth is, the product can contain up to 0.5 gram of trans fats and still claim to be trans fat–free, because, as we noted in Sample 2, the FDA says manufacturers can round down the figures on the Nutrition Facts panels.

Sample 4

You may see the following label:

- Total fat: 4 grams
- Saturated fat: 0.5 gram

This is a label for a brand of flour tortillas. You don't know the identity of the missing 3.5 grams of fat: They could be polyunsaturated, monounsaturated, and/or trans fats—in any combination. Your next step is to look at the ingredient list to see if the words "partially hydrogenated vegetable oil" or "shortening" appear. For this product, the first three ingredients on the label are "enriched flour, water, liquid soybean oil," but there is no listing for partially hydrogenated vegetable oil. Liquid soybean oil contains a high percentage of polyunsaturated fat (61 percent) and a respectable amount of monounsaturated fat (24 percent), and only 15 percent saturated fat (see chart, "Breakdown of Fats in Different Oils" on page 19).

Chances are good that the 3.5 grams of missing fat are polyunsaturated and monounsaturated.

Sample 5

Let's look at a label for a brand of barbecue potato chips:

- Total fat: 10 grams
- Saturated fat: 2.5 grams

Immediately you notice the big discrepancy between the total fat and saturated fat: 7.5 grams. One look at the ingredient list tells you the story: "potatoes, vegetable oil (may contain one or more of the following: cottonseed, corn, canola, sunflower, partially hydrogenated [cottonseed or corn] oil), salt," and so on. The partially hydrogenated oils are the second ingredient, so you can be sure that the majority of the 7.5 grams is trans fats.

Sample 6

You may also find labels like the following one for a can of black olives:

- Total fat: 2.5 grams
- Monounsaturated fat: 1.5 grams
- Polyunsaturated fat: 0 grams

If you're wondering where the information for saturated fat is (which is required), the manufacturer has added a footnote to the label, which reads "Not a significant source of saturated fat." That means the amount of saturated fat in the olives is less than 0.5 gram per serving. The missing 1 gram of fat is thus divided up between polyunsaturated (even though the label says 0 grams, anything less than 0.5 gram can be stated as 0) and saturated fats. Because there is no partially hydrogenated vegetable oil in the ingredient list, trans fats are not present.

Sample 7

Here's a label that can make you stop and think for a few minutes: one for a natural peanut butter, Laura Scudders:

- Total fat: 16 grams
- Saturated fat: 2 grams

At first glance, you notice that there are 14 grams of fat unaccounted for—a large amount. But inspection of the ingredient list shows that the only ingredients are peanuts and salt—no hydrogenated or partially hydrogenated oils or shortening. Thus there are no trans fats in this food. A call to the manufacturer confirms what you've concluded, and the consumer information department reveals that the remaining 14 grams consist of 8 grams monounsaturated fat and 6 grams polyunsaturated fat.

GENERAL GUIDELINES FOR READING FOOD LABELS

Here are some general tips to remember when you read Nutrition Facts panels and ingredient lists. These guidelines will come in handy when you go shopping and when you're using products you already have at home. You might want to keep this list with you while you shop or post it on your refrigerator until the guidelines become a regular part of your shopping habit. The instructions in the box, "How to Read Nutrition Facts Panels" on page 37, can also help you read food labels for trans fat content.

- Consider both the Nutrition Facts panel and the ingredient list when trying to identify the amount of trans fats in a product.
- When reading the ingredient lists, if you see the words "partially hydrogenated vegetable shortening," "partially hydrogenated vegetable oil," "shortening," or "margarine" near the top of the list, the product contains a significant amount of trans fats. If the words appear near the bottom of the list, the amount of trans fats is likely to be much less.
- Check serving sizes. If one serving of your favorite cookie contains only 1 gram of trans fats and 1 gram of saturated fats and you eat only one cookie, then your total combined trans and saturated fat intake is only 2 grams. But if you normally eat five or six cookies a day, then your total daily consumption of combined trans fats and saturated fats is 10 to 12 grams.

- Foods that are low in total fat are probably also low in trans fats. The higher the amount of saturated fats in a product, the more likely there is a significant amount of trans fats as well.

- Packages that say "contains no saturated fat" or "saturated fat free" contain less than 0.5 gram of saturated fat and less than 0.5 gram of trans fats per serving. That means, if each serving actually contains 0.4 gram of saturated or trans fats and you eat two or three servings, you've consumed 0.8 to 1.2 grams of fat. This is not a large amount of fat, but if you are eating several different foods with "hidden" fats, then the accumulation of these fats could be significant.

- Labels that say "low saturated fat" may still contain a significant amount of trans fats. Check the Nutrition Facts panel and ingredients.

- Know what's really behind a manufacturer's claims. "Fat-free" means that each serving of the product contains less than 0.5 gram of fat per serving; "low-fat" means there are 3 grams or less per serving; and "low-saturated fat" means there is 1 gram or less per serving.

- Similarly, do not be fooled by words on the package such as "healthy," "light," or "nutritious." "Healthy" and "nutritious" as compared with what? "Light" can mean light in color or in weight and have nothing to do with the fat content. Always read the Nutrition Facts panel and the ingredients list.

- Foods that should send up a red flag include anything that is deep fried, snack foods (e.g., potato and tortilla chips, rinds), crackers, and commercial baked goods.

- Avoid hard margarines. If you want to use margarine, use a soft brand that comes in a tub. Better yet, avoid all margarines—and butter, which doesn't have trans fats but is high in saturated fats—and use olive oil on bread or a fat substitute for baking (see chapter 6 for fat substitutions).

HOW TO READ NUTRITION FACTS PANELS

If the trans fat level is given:

- If 0 grams, check the saturated fat level to see how it contributes to the daily level of fat considered to be healthy for you.
- If the product contains trans fats, decide if the amount per serving (or the number of servings you plan to eat) fits into the daily total of saturated and trans fats considered to be healthy for you.

If the trans fat level is not given, read the ingredient list:

- If the ingredient list shows hydrogenated or partially hydrogenated oil and/or shortening/margarine, check the amount of total fat, satu-

---

rated fat, and, if provided, polyunsaturated and monounsaturated fat levels as well to help you determine the amount of trans fats in the item. *Remember*: The higher on the list hydrogenated or partially hydrogenated oil and/or shortening/margarine are on the list, the higher the amount of trans fats in the food.

- If the ingredient list does not show hydrogenated or partially hydrogenated oil and/or shortening/margarine, check the amounts of total and saturated fats in the food to see how they contribute to the daily levels considered to be healthy for you.

GETTING INFORMATION FROM FOOD MANUFACTURERS

It's important for you to know that you can contact the manufacturer of any food product and ask questions about nutritional values, ingredients, and other concerns. Many manufacturers make it easy for you: There's often a toll-free customer service number on the packaging. Some producers supply only their address, which means you'll have to do some investigating to find them. Occasionally you'll see a Web site address on labels as well. If you have Internet access, you can search for food manufacturers online and explore their Web sites for information on nutrition and ingredients. Contact information—telephone numbers, fax, e-mail address, physical address—is typically provided as well. See the Appendix for contact information for some of the most common food manufacturers in the United States.

If you call the customer service number for a food manufacturer, the individual who answers the phone may not be able to give you the information you request. In that case, ask to be transferred to a product information specialist. Of all the manufacturers we contacted, all were more than happy to supply the information requested.

BOTTOM LINE

In this chapter you learned how to determine how many grams of trans and saturated fats are considered to be safe and healthy for you. You also learned how to decipher food labels so you can identify the amount of trans fats in any given item. As time goes on, this task will become increasingly easier, as you become familiar with the foods that have little or no trans fats, and as more and more food manufacturers list the trans fat levels on their products.

CHAPTER 4

How to Eat at Fast-Food and Other Restaurants

According to the National Restaurant Association, the average American aged eight years and older eats an average of 4.2 commercially prepared meals per week. Chances are, you or someone you know eats away from home even more often: In fact, men ages twenty-five to thirty-four eat out an average of six times per week. Lunch is the meal Americans eat out most often, and the choice of food establishments is likely to be fast food (e.g., McDonald's, Wendy's, Taco Bell) or a family restaurant chain (e.g., Applebee's, T.G.I. Friday's, Village Inn).

Although convenience is the number one reason people eat out, you may be sacrificing your health in the process. At home, you have control over the amount of trans fats and saturated fats in the foods you prepare and serve; yet that certainty disappears when you eat at a restaurant. Restaurants are not required to list the amount of trans fats in the foods they serve. In fact, can you think of a time when you went to a restaurant and you saw the nutritional information listed for the foods you ordered? We're sure your fast-food chicken sandwich doesn't come in a box that says "26 grams fat, 15 grams saturated fat, 3 grams trans fat, 4 grams polyunsaturated fat, 4 grams monounsaturated fat."

The truth is, you won't know any of the nutritional information about the food you buy in a restaurant unless you ask about each item you order (and then hope the information is accurate), or you go to the restaurant's Web site, if it has one, and look for nutritional information there, or you contact the restaurant's consumer relations department and ask for specific nutritional information. Naturally, none of these options is convenient.

This chapter hopes to make this task a lot easier. In the pages that follow, we look at some of the fast-food restaurants and the more popular items on their menus, list the amount of fats they contain, and indicate whether they are prepared with and/or contain partially hydrogenated vegetable oil or shortening. We also show you a list of Best Bets items at each establishment. The first criterion for a Best Bet was that it not contain (to the best of our knowledge) any hydrogenated/partially hydrogenated fats. If it passed that test, we looked at the total fat compared with saturated fat. Generally, saturated fat levels of 2 grams or less were acceptable, with a moderate total fat level of 5 grams. Please note that Best Bets are not necessarily healthy choices: They may contain, depending on the food item, unhealthy amounts of white flour, sugar, salt, and food additives. Your *real* best bet is to skip the fast-food restaurants and prepare wholesome meals at home or go to a restaurant that serves natural, whole foods or has a heart-healthy menu.

For individuals who dine at more formal restaurants, this chapter also looks at different classifications of foods (e.g., Italian, Mexican, Oriental/Eastern, Indian/Middle Eastern, vegetarian, seafood) and offers some general guidelines on which foods are most likely to contain trans fats and which questions to ask your servers and food preparers to ensure you get healthy foods in such restaurants.

FAST-FOOD RESTAURANTS

The following lists provide nutritional information on some of the popular items served at fast-food restaurants across the United States. Not all items are available in all restaurants in all areas, and actual fat content may be slightly different from location to location. Restaurants are not required to provide trans fat information; however, one of them has provided it. In all cases, we tell you the total fat and saturated fat levels in grams, and, when the information is available, whether the item contains and/or is cooked in hydrogenated or partially hydrogenated oils or shortening.

Restaurants may change their ingredients and/or methods of food preparation at any time. That's why it's important for you to ask questions about the food you order. Although some fast-food establishments may say you can get your food the way you want it, chances are no one is going to bake french fries for you or order special shortening-free biscuits for your breakfast sandwich.

Note: We have relied on information provided by the restaurants on their Web sites. All information is per serving. In the "Trans Fat" column, a "Y" indicates that the item contains an undisclosed amount of trans fats based on information that one or more of the ingredients contains hydrogenated or partially hydrogenated oils or shortening, and/or is cooked in them; "P" indicates that the item probably or possibly contains trans fats; and "NA" means no information was available to make a determination. See the Appendix for these restaurants' contact information.

Arby's

Note: All fried foods are cooked in 100 percent corn oil. However, the oil used to toast the buns is partially hydrogenated. Not all Arby's locations use this oil. The following items contain hydrogenated or partially hydrogenated oil: biscuits, cheddar cheese sauce, grilled chicken, chocolate syrup, seasoned croutons, seasoned curly fries, egg patty, homestyle fries, Italian Parmesan dressing, jalapeño bites, mozzarella sticks, multigrain buns, onion petals, onion rolls, roast chicken breast, sesame seed bun, sub rolls.

THE TRANS FAT REMEDY

Arby's (cont.)

	Total Fat	Sat. Fat	Trans Fat
Sandwiches			
Arby-Q	14	4	Y
Beef 'N Cheddar	24	8	Y
Big Montana	32	15	Y
Chicken Bacon 'N Swiss	33	8	Y
Chicken Breast Fillet	30	5	Y
Chicken Cordon Bleu	35	8	Y
Giant Roast Beef	23	10	Y
Grilled Chicken Deluxe	22	4	Y
Junior Roast Beef	13	4.5	Y
Melt w/Cheddar	15	5	Y
Regular Roast Beef	16	6	Y
Subs			
French Dip	18	8	Y
Ham 'N Swiss	27	8	Y
Italian	53	15	Y
Philly Beef 'N Swiss	42	15	Y
Roast Beef	48	16	Y
Turkey	37	9	Y
Breakfast			
Biscuit w/ham	20	5	Y
Biscuit w/sausage	33	9	Y
Biscuit w/bacon	21	5	Y
Croissant w/ham	19	11	Y
Croissant w/sausage	32	15	Y
Croissant w/bacon	20	11	Y
Sides and Salads			
Caesar Salad, no dressing	4	2.5	NA
Cheddar Curly Fries	24	6	Y

Arby's (cont.)

	Total Fat	Sat. Fat	Trans Fat
Chicken Fingers, 4-pack	38	8	Y
Chicken Finger Salad, no dressing	34	9	NA
Curly Fries:			
Small	15	3.5	Y
Medium	20	5	Y
Large	30	7	Y
Grilled Chicken Caesar, no dressing	8	3.5	Y
Homestyle Fries:			
Small	13	3.5	Y
Medium	16	4	Y
Large	24	6	Y
Jalapeno Bites	21	9	Y
Mozzarella Sticks (4)	29	14	Y
Onion Petals	24	3.5	Y
Turkey Club Salad, no dressing	21	10	NA
Sauces			
BBQ Dipping	0	0	NA
Blue Cheese	31	6	NA
Buttermilk Ranch	30	5	NA
Honey French	24	4	NA
Honey Mustard	12	1.5	NA
Italian Parmesan	24	4	NA
Tangy Southwest Sauce	26	4.5	NA
Thousand Island	28	4.5	NA

BEST BETS: Caesar Salad, no dressing

THE TRANS FAT REMEDY

Boston Market

	Total Fat	Sat. Fat	Trans Fat
Entrées			
¼ White Meat Chicken, no wing or skin	4	1	NA
¼ White Meat Chicken, w/skin and wing	12	3.5	NA
¼ Dark Meat Chicken, no skin	10	3	NA
¼ Dark Meat Chicken, w/skin	21	6	NA
½ Chicken w/skin	33	10	NA
Grilled Chicken, BBQ	19	7	NA
Grilled Chicken, Teriyaki	10	2	NA
Honey Glazed Ham	8	3	NA
Meat Loaf w/tomato sauce	19	8	NA
Marinated Grilled Chicken	10	2	NA
Pastry Top Chicken Pot Pie	46	14	Y
Pastry Top Turkey Pot Pie	41	13	Y
Sides, Soups, Salads			
Butternut Squash	6	4	NA
Caesar Side Salad	26	4.5	P
Chicken Gravy	0.5	0	NA
Chicken Tortilla Soup, w/toppings	8	2.5	P
Chunky Chicken Salad	39	6	P
Homestyle Mashed Potatoes	9	5	P
Macaroni and Cheese	11	6	P

Boston Market (cont.)

	Total Fat	Sat. Fat	Trans Fat
Oriental Grilled Chicken Salad, w/dressing & noodles	24	3.5	Y
Rice Pilaf	4	0.5	NA
Southwest Grilled Chicken Salad, w/dressing & chips	58	11	Y
Stuffing	8	1.5	P
Steamed Vegetable Medley	0	0	NA
Tortellini Salad	24	6	P
Turkey Tortilla Soup, w/toppings	7	2	P
Sandwiches			
BBQ Grilled Chicken	45	11	Y
Chicken, w/cheese & sauce	29	7	Y
Chicken, no cheese or sauce	6	0.5	Y
Marinated Grilled Chicken	36	6	Y
Teriyaki Grilled Chicken	26	4.5	Y
Turkey Bacon Club	37	12	Y
Desserts			
Apple Streusel Pie	15	3	Y
Cherry Streusel Pie	14	3	Y
Chocolate Cake	32	8	Y
Chocolate Chip Cookie	19	6	Y
Hummingbird Cake	36	14	Y

BEST BETS: ¼ white chicken (no wing or skin), chicken gravy, rice pilaf, steamed vegetable medley

Burger King

Note: The following items or ingredients used at Burger King contain partially hydrogenated oil: grilled patties, 4" and 5" buns, specialty buns, chicken breast fillets for Chicken Whopper and Jr. version, breaded chicken patty, chicken tenders, fish, egg patty, puffy scrambled egg patty, vanilla bean cheesecake, croutons, creamy caesar dressing, sausage, croissant, Cini-Minis, French toast sticks, french fries, onion rings, hash brown rounds, Dutch apple pie, Hershey's sundae pie, hot fudge brownie royale, Nestlé Toll House chocolate chip cookies.

	Total Fat	Sat. Fat	Trans Fat
Sandwiches			
Bacon Cheeseburger	20	9	0.6
Bacon Double Cheeseburger	34	17	1.3
BK Veggie	10	1.5	0.1
Cheeseburger	17	8	0.7
Double Whopper	62	22	1.9
Double Whopper w/cheese	70	27	2.1
Hamburger	13	5	0.5
King Supreme	34	14	1.2
Whopper	43	13	1.0
Whopper w/cheese	50	18	1.4
Whopper Jr.	22	7	0.5
Whopper Jr. w/cheese	26	9	0.7
Chicken and Fish			
Fish Filet	30	8	0.4

Burger King (cont.)

	Total Fat	Sat. Fat	Trans Fat
Chicken Whopper	26	5	0.5
Chicken Whopper Jr.	14	2.5	0.3
Chicken Specialty	28	6	2.2
Chicken Tenders:			
4 pieces	9	2.5	2.0
6 pieces	14	4	2.7
8 pieces	19	5	3.6

Sides

	Total Fat	Sat. Fat	Trans Fat
Chili	8	3	0.3
French Fries:			
Small	11	3	3.0
Value	17	4.5	4.4
Medium	18	5	4.7
Large	25	7	6.4
King	30	8	7.8
Onion Rings:			
Small	9	2	2.0
Value	13	3.5	3.1
Medium	16	4	3.6
Large	23	6	5.4
King	27	7	6.0

Breakfast

	Total Fat	Sat. Fat	Trans Fat
Croissan'wich, w/sausage, egg & cheese	39	14	2.5
Croissan'wich w/sausage & cheese	31	11	2.4
Croissan'wich w/egg & cheese	19	7	1.9
French Toast Sticks (5)	20	4.5	4.5

Burger King (cont.)

	Total Fat	Sat. Fat	Trans Fat
Hash Brown Rounds:			
Small	15	4	4.9
Large	25	7	8.4
Sourdough Breakfast Sandwich, w/sausage, egg & cheese	39	13	0.9
Sourdough Breakfast Sandwich, w/bacon, egg & cheese	22	8	0.3
Sourdough Breakfast Sandwich, w/ham, egg & cheese	20	7	0.3
Desserts			
Dutch Apple Pie	14	3	3.0
Hershey's Sundae Pie	18	10	1.5
Ice Cream Shakes:			
Vanilla, value	24	16	1.1
Vanilla, small	32	21	2.0
Vanilla, medium	41	27	2.0
Chocolate, small	32	21	2.0
Chocolate, medium	42	27	2.0
Strawberry, small	32	21	2.0
Strawberry, medium	41	27	2.0
Nestlé Toll House Cookies (2)	16	5	0.4

BEST BETS: BK Veggie, with reservation, because the total fat content is 10. However, the trans fat and saturated fat levels are acceptable.

Dairy Queen

	Total Fat	Sat. Fat	Trans Fat
Ice Cream Treats			
Banana Split	12	8	NA
Buster Bar	28	12	NA
Chocolate Dilly Bar	13	7	NA
DQ Sandwich	6	3	NA
DQ Fudge Bar, no added sugar	0	0	NA
Oreo Cookies Blizzard:			
Small	18	9	NA
Medium	23	11	NA
Chocolate Chip Cookie Dough Blizzard:			
Small	24	13	NA
Medium	36	19	NA
Cone, vanilla:			
Small	7	4.5	NA
Medium	9	6	NA
Large	12	8	NA
Cone, chocolate:			
Small	8	5	NA
Medium	11	7	NA
Dipped cone:			
Small	17	9	NA
Medium	24	13	NA
Heath DQ Treatzza Pizza	7	3.5	NA
Malt, small chocolate	16	10	NA
Misty Slush, small	0	0	NA
M&M DQ Treatzza Pizza	7	4	NA
Peanut Buster Parfait	31	17	NA

Dairy Queen (cont.)

	Total Fat	Sat. Fat	Trans Fat
Pecan Mudslide Treat	30	12	NA
Shake, small chocolate	15	10	NA
Soft Serve, vanilla cup	4.5	3	NA
Soft Serve, chocolate cup	5	3.5	NA
Soft Serve, vanilla cone:			
Small	7	4.5	NA
Medium	9	6	NA
Large	12	8	NA
Soft Serve, chocolate cone:			
Small	8	5	NA
Medium	11	7	NA
Sandwiches and Sides			
Chicken Breast Fillet			
Sandwich	10	2.5	NA
Grilled Chicken Salad	32	8	NA
Chicken Strip Basket	50	13	NA
Chili 'N' Cheese Dog	21	9	NA
Crispy Chicken Salad	51	11	NA
French Fries:			
Small	18	3.5	NA
Medium	23	4.5	NA
DQ Homestyle Hamburger	12	5	NA
DQ Homestyle			
Cheeseburger	17	8	NA
DQ Homestyle Double			
Cheeseburger	31	16	NA
DQ Homestyle Bacon			
Double Cheeseburger	36	18	NA
Hot Dog	14	5	NA

Dairy Queen (cont.)

	Total Fat	Sat. Fat	Trans Fat
Onion Rings	16	4	NA
DQ Ultimate Burger	43	19	NA

BEST BETS: DQ Fudge Bar and Misty Slush

Jack in the Box

Note: The following items contain partially hydrogenated oils; those marked with (#) are also cooked in oil: apple turnover, biscuits, cheesecake, cheese sauce, cheese sticks#, chicken breast pieces#, chicken fajita patty, chicken patty, spicy chicken breast fillet, creamy Southwest dressing, croissants, croutons, double fudge cake, grilled egg#, egg rolls#, fish#, french fries#, French toast sticks#, guacamole, hash browns#, onion rings#, Oreo cookie crumbs, Philly beef steak, potato wedges#, seasoned curly fries#, sourdough bread, Southwest chicken salad, stuffed jalapeños#, tacos, Monster tacos, taquito (cooked shredded beef), wonton strips. The buns do *not* contain partially hydrogenated oil.

	Total Fat	Sat. Fat	Trans Fat
Sandwiches			
Bacon Bacon Cheeseburger	59	19	NA
Bacon Ultimate Cheeseburger	75	28	NA
Big Cheeseburger	40	16	NA
Chili Cheeseburger	20	9	NA

Jack in the Box (cont.)

	Total Fat	Sat. Fat	Trans Fat
Hamburger	14	6	NA
Jumbo Jack	31	11	NA
Jumbo Jack w/cheese	38	16	NA
Philly Cheesesteak	22	11	Y
Sourdough Jack	49	16	Y
Turkey Jack	32	11	NA
Ultimate Cheeseburger	66	28	NA
Chicken and Fish Items			
Chicken Breast Pieces (5)	17	3	Y
Chicken Fajita Pita	11	4.5	Y
Chicken Sandwich	21	4.5	Y
Fish & Chips	31	7	Y
Jack's Spicy Chicken	37	10	Y
Sourdough Grilled Chicken			
Club	28	6	P
Sides			
Bacon Cheddar Potato			
Wedges	53	16	Y
Cheese Sticks (3)	12	5	Y
Chili Cheese Curly Fries	40	11	Y
French Fries:			
Small	16	3.5	Y
Large	28	6	Y
Monster Taco	15	5	Y
Onion Rings	30	5	Y
Seasoned Curly Fries	23	5	Y
Taco	9	3	Y
Tacquitos (3)	17	7	Y
Breakfast			
Breakfast Jack	14	5	P

Jack in the Box (cont.)

	Total Fat	Sat. Fat	Trans Fat
Extreme Sausage			
Sandwich	53	18	P
French Toast Sticks (4)	18	4	Y
Hash Browns	10	2.5	Y
Sausage Biscuit	27	8	Y
Sausage Croissant	50	15	Y
Sausage, Egg & Cheese			
Biscuit	60	20	Y
Sourdough Breakfast			
Sandwich	26	8	Y
Supreme Croissant	37	9	Y
Salads			
Asian Chicken	35.5	5	P
Chicken Club	65	13	P
Southwest Chicken,			
w/dressing	44	11	Y

BEST BETS: None

KFC (Kentucky Fried Chicken)

Note: All chicken and potatoes are cooked in oil.

	Total Fat	Sat. Fat	Trans Fat
Entrées			
Chicken Pot Pie	40	15	Y
EC (Extra Crispy)			
Chicken, Breast	28	8	Y
EC Chicken, Thigh	26	7	Y

KFC (cont.)

	Total Fat	Sat. Fat	Trans Fat
EC Chicken, Drumstick	10	2.5	Y
Hot and Spicy, Breast	27	8	Y
Hot and Spicy, Drumstick	9	2.5	Y
Hot and Spicy, Thigh	28	8	Y
Popcorn Chicken:			
Individual	30	7	Y
Kids	18	4	Y
Large	44	10	Y
Sandwiches			
HBBQ Sandwich	6	1.5	NA
OR (Original Recipe) Sandwich, w/sauce	27	6	Y
OR Sandwich, no sauce	13	4	Y
TC (Triple Crunch) Sandwich, w/sauce	40	8	Y
TC Sandwich, no sauce	26	6	Y
TR (Tender Roast) Sandwich, w/sauce	19	4	Y
TR Sandwich, no sauce	5	1.5	Y
Twister	38	7	Y
Zinger, w/sauce	41	8	Y
Other Items			
Biscuit, w/gravy	10	2	Y
Cole Slaw	11	2	NA
Crispy Strips (6)	24	5	Y
HBBQ Wings (6)	33	7	Y
Hot Wings (6)	29	6	Y
Macaroni and Cheese	6	2	NA

KFC (cont.)

	Total Fat	Sat. Fat	Trans Fat
Mashed potatoes, w/gravy	4.5	1	NA
Potato Wedges	12	3	Y
Desserts			
Apple Pie	9	2	P
Lemon Meringue Pie	11	5	P
Lil' Bucket, chocolate cream	13	8	NA
Lil' Bucket, fudge brownie	9	4	P
Lil' Bucket, lemon cream	14	7	P
Lil' Bucket, strawberry shortcake	6	4	P
Pecan Pie	15	2.5	P

BEST BETS: Mashed potatoes with gravy. Your real best bet is to try one of the potato recipes and gravy recipes in chapter 6.

. Pizza Hut

Note: The following items contain partially hydrogenated oil: dessert pizza (thin crust), alfredo sauce, white pasta sauce, cooked diced chicken, meatballs, crumb topping. The hand-tossed, pan, and stuffed crust pizza crusts may contain partially hydrogenated oil. Both the mild and hot wings are cooked in partially hydrogenated oil. Also note that slice sizes vary considerably, depending on the pie you order.

Pizza Hut (cont.)

	Total Fat	Sat. Fat	Trans Fat
P'zone Pizza (1 serving = ½ P'zone)			
Classic	23	12	NA
Meat Lover's	31	15	P
Pepperoni	24	12	NA
Hand-Tossed (1 slice)			
Beef	17	8	P
Cheese	10	5	P
Chicken Supreme	7	3.5	P
Meat Lover's	17	7	P
Pepperoni Lover's	11	4.5	P
Pepperoni	13	6	P
Pork	16	7	P
Sausage	18	8	P
Supreme	12	5	P
Super Supreme	14	6	P
Veggie Lover's	8	3	P
Chicago Dish			
Meat Lover's	27	12	P
Pepperoni	20	9	NA
Pepperoni, Sausage &			
Mushroom	22	10	NA
Supreme	23	10	NA
Veggie Lover's	18	8	NA
Stuffed Crust Gold			
Beef	24	13	P
Cheese	20	11	P
Chicken Supreme	18	10	P
Diced Chicken	18	10	P
Meat Lover's	29	14	P

Pizza Hut (cont.)

	Total Fat	Sat. Fat	Trans Fat
Pepperoni	20	10	P
Pepperoni Lover's	25	13	P
Sausage Lover's	27	13	P
Sausage	27	13	P
Supreme	24	12	P
Super Supreme	26	13	P
Veggie Lover's	18	9	P
Personal Pan (1 serving = 1 pizza)			
Beef	35	14	Y
Cheese	28	12	Y
Pepperoni	28	11	Y
Pork	34	13	Y
Sausage	39	14	Y
Pan (1 serving = 1 slice)			
Beef	18	7	P
Cheese	14	6	P
Chicken Supreme	12	4	P
Meat Lover's	21	7	P
Pepperoni	14	5	P
Pepperoni Lover's	18	7	P
Sausage	20	7	P
Supreme	17	6	P
Super Supreme	18	6	P
Veggie Lover's	12	4	P
Sandwiches			
Ham and cheese	21	7	NA
Supreme Sandwich	28	10	NA

Pizza Hut (cont.)

	Total Fat	Sat. Fat	Trans Fat
Appetizers			
Beef Wings, mild	12	3.5	Y
Beef Wings, hot	12	3	Y
Breadstick	4	1	NA
Garlic Bread	8	1.5	NA
Sauces/Dressings			
Blue Cheese	14	3	NA
Beef Wing Blue Cheese Dip	24	4	NA
Beef Wing Ranch	24	4	NA
Creamy Caesar	15	2.5	NA
Creamy Cucumber, low calorie	7	1	NA
Garlic Parmesan Mayo Dressing	21	3	NA
Desserts			
Apple Dessert Pizza (1 slice)	4.5	1	Y
Cherry Dessert Pizza	4.5	1	Y
Cinnamon Sticks (2)	5	1	NA

BEST BETS: None. Stay at home and make your own pizza (see recipe in chapter 6).

Subway

Note: The following breads used at Subway contain partially hydrogenated oil: Italian, Parmesan/Oregano, Roasted Garlic, Italian Herb & Cheese. Thus, depending on which bread you request for your sandwich, your meal may contain trans fats, so all sandwiches have a "P" rating in the trans fat column. The following items contain partially hydrogenated oil: chicken breast patty, meatballs, all cookies. All sauces and dressings are trans fat–free.

	Total Fat	Sat. Fat	Trans Fat
Sandwiches (all 6")			
BMT	24	9	P
Chicken Pizziola	16	6	P
Dijon Horseradish Melt	21	7	P
Honey Mustard Ham	5	1.5	P
Meatball	26	11	P
Steak & Cheese	14	5	P
Subway Melt	15	6	P
Sweet Onion Chicken Teriyaki	5	1.5	P
Southwest Turkey Bacon	16	4.5	P
Southwest Steak & Cheese	19	6	P
Subway Club	6	2	P
Turkey Breast	4.5	1.5	P
Veggie Delite	3	1	P
Deli Sandwiches			
Ham	4	1.5	P
Roast Beef	4.5	2	P
Tuna	16	4.5	P
Turkey Breast	3.5	1.5	P
Breakfast Sandwiches			
Bacon & Egg	15	4.5	P
Cheese & Egg	15	5	P
Ham & Egg	13	3.5	P
Western Egg	12	3.5	P

Subway (cont.)

Salads	Total Fat	Sat. Fat	Trans Fat
BMT	19	8	NA
Meatball	20	10	Y
Melt	10	4.5	NA
Roast Chicken Breast	3	1	NA
Seafood & Crab	11	3.5	NA
Tuna	16	4	NA
Veggie Delite	1	1	NA
Soups			
Black Bean	4.5	2	NA
Broccoli Cheese	12	4	NA
Chicken Dumpling	4.5	2.5	NA
Chili	14	5	NA
Cream of Potato w/Bacon	12	4	NA
Minestrone	1	0	NA
Roast Chicken Noodle	4	1	NA
Vegetable Beef	1.5	0.5	NA
Cookies			
Chocolate Chip	10	4	Y
M&M	10	4	Y
Oatmeal Raisin	8	2.5	Y
Peanut Butter	12	4	Y
Fruizles (all)	0	0	NA

BEST BETS: Veggie Delite and roast chicken breast salads; minestrone soup; black bean soup; roast chicken noodle soup; vegetable beef soup; all Fruizles

Taco Bell

Note: Chalupas and gorditas are made with flat bread, which is free of partially hydrogenated oil; however, chalupas are fried in oil and gorditas are not. The tortillas used for burritos and quesadillas contain partially hydrogenated oil.

	Total Fat	Sat. Fat	Trans Fat
Chalupas			
Baja, steak	25	7	Y
Baja, beef	27	8	Y
Baja, chicken	24	6	Y
Nacho Cheese, chicken	18	5	Y
Nacho Cheese, beef	22	7	Y
Nacho Cheese, steak	19	5	Y
Supreme, beef	24	10	Y
Supreme, chicken	20	8	Y
Supreme, steak	22	8	Y
Burritos			
Bean	10	3.5	Y
Chili Cheese	18	9	Y
Fiesta, beef	15	5	Y
Fiesta, chicken	12	3.5	Y
Fiesta, steak	13	4	Y
Grilled Stuft, beef	33	11	Y
Grilled Stuft, chicken	26	7	Y
Grilled Stuft, steak	28	8	Y
7-Layer	22	8	Y
Supreme, beef	18	8	Y
Supreme, chicken	14	6	Y
Supreme, steak	16	7	Y

Taco Bell (cont.)

	Total Fat	Sat. Fat	Trans Fat
Gorditas			
Baja, beef	19	5	P
Baja, chicken	15	3.5	P
Nacho Cheese, beef	13	4	P
Nacho Cheese, chicken	10	2.5	P
Nacho Cheese, steak	11	3	P
Breakfast			
Burrito	25	9	Y
Gordita	24	7	P
Quesadilla	20	9	Y
Steak Burrito	26	10	Y
Steak Quesadilla	23	10	Y
Tacos			
Double Decker	14	5	P
Double Decker Supreme	18	8	P
Grilled Steak Soft Taco	17	4.5	P
Soft, beef	10	4.5	P
Soft, chicken	6	2.5	P
Soft Supreme, beef	14	7	P
Soft Supreme, chicken	10	5	P
Taco	10	4	P
Taco Supreme	14	7	P
Other Items			
Cheese Quesadilla	28	13	Y
Chicken Quesadilla	30	13	Y
Mexican Pizza	31	11	P
Nachos BellGrande	43	13	P
Nachos Supreme	26	9	P
Southwest Steak Bowl	32	8	Y

Taco Bell (cont.)

	Total Fat	Sat. Fat	Trans Fat
Taco Salad with Salsa	42	15	Y
Zesty Chicken Border Bowl	42	9	Y

BEST BETS: None. Try the Potato Enchilada recipe in chapter 6, or make your own burritos using low-fat flour tortillas, low-fat refried beans, vegetable toppings, and salsa.

Wendy's

Note: The french fries contain and are cooked in hydrogenated oil. All the buns contain partially hydrogenated oil, and all chicken items except the grilled chicken are cooked in partially hydrogenated oil. However, the grilled chicken contains partially hydrogenated oil.

	Total Fat	Sat. Fat	Trans Fat
Sandwiches			
Big Bacon Classic	29	12	Y
Chicken Breast Fillet	16	3	Y
Chicken Club	19	4	Y
Classic Single w/everything	19	7	Y
Grilled Chicken	7	1.5	Y
Jr. Hamburger	9	3	Y
Jr. Cheeseburger	12	5	Y
Jr. Bacon Cheeseburger	18	7	Y
Jr. Cheeseburger Deluxe	16	6	Y
Spicy Chicken	15	3	Y

THE TRANS FAT REMEDY

Wendy's (cont.)

Salads	Total Fat	Sat. Fat	Trans Fat
Caesar side, w/croutons & dressing	22.5	4.5	P
Side Salad	0	0	NA
Chicken BLT Salad, w/croutons & dressing	44.5	12	P
Mandarin chicken salad, w/nuts, noodles & dressing	33	4	P
Spring Mix Salad, w/nuts & dressing	42	9.5	P
Taco Supreme Salad, w/chips, sour cream & salsa	34	14.5	P
Other Items			
Crispy Chicken Nuggets:			
5-piece	14	3	Y
4-piece, kids'	11	2.5	Y
Honey Mustard Sauce	12	2	NA
French Fries:			
Kids	11	2	Y
Medium	17	3	Y
Biggie	19	3.5	Y
Great Biggie	23	4.5	Y
Frosty:			
Junior	4	2.5	NA
Small	8	5	NA
Medium	11	7	NA

Wendy's (cont.)

	Total Fat	Sat. Fat	Trans Fat
Hot Stuffed Baked Potato:			
Plain	0	0	NA
Bacon & Cheese	22	6	NA
Broccoli & Cheese	14	3	NA

BEST BETS: Side salad, plain baked potato. Your real best bet is to try some of the delicious recipes in chapter 6, including the Stuffed Baked Potato.

DINING OUT IN OTHER RESTAURANTS

When eating out in restaurants other than fast-food establishments, you have a bit more control over how your food is prepared and what ingredients are used, within reason. If a restaurant only has breads that contain partially hydrogenated oils, you can't expect the chef to run out and purchase special bread just for you. Your choice at that moment is to either skip the bread or not. However, if you voice your opinions about healthier breads, you may see them on the menu on your next visit.

The same may be true for food preparation. If the menu says "fried flounder" and you want the cook to bake it for you, you may or may not get your request, depending on the restaurant. If all the restaurant's fish is supplied to them already breaded and prefried and all the cook does is quick-fry it, avoiding trans fats isn't possible. However, if the fish is fresh and the cook is willing to prepare your dish baked even though it isn't on the menu, then you get it your way. Some restaurants print on their menus "No substitutions," which may mean they won't prepare an item differently from how it's listed on the menu.

All that being said, here are some guidelines for avoiding trans fats when eating out at various types of restaurants. *Bon appétit!*

Italian Restaurants/Pizzerias

- Before you take a bite of that crusty Italian bread, ask your server for a list of the ingredients. If you do decide to order the bread, ask for olive oil on the side instead of margarine.
- Skip anything fried—calamari, mushrooms, fish, mozzarella sticks, veal—if it's been prepared in partially hydrogenated oil or shortening. Ask your server. If you want to reduce your intake of saturated fat, avoid anything that is fried. A tip-off on the menu is the word "*frito*," which means "fried."
- Ask if the cook fries or sautés the meats (including meatballs) in partially hydrogenated oil. Avoid any entrée that contains those items.
- The right sauce can make the meal, but you need to know what's in the one you choose. Red sauces are generally free of trans fats, but you should still ask your server about the ingredients. White sauces (e.g., alfredo, white clam, white garlic), however, are more likely to contain partially

hydrogenated oils. White sauces are also usually very high in saturated fat.

- Pizza crust may contain partially hydrogenated oils, especially if prepared commercially. If the restaurant makes its own crust, ask what ingredients are used.

- When it comes to salad dressings, oil and vinegar and herbed oils are safe. Creamy dressings are more likely to contain partially hydrogenated oils. If you really want a creamy dressing, why not bring your own from home (see our recipes in chapter 6).

- Cakes, pies, and cookies are havens for partially hydrogenated oils. If the restaurant makes its own desserts, it's possible the baker uses butter only. Ask your server. You can always pass on the baked goods and opt for sorbet, spumoni, or Italian ice.

Oriental/Eastern

- "Fried," "crispy," and "tempura" are the words you are looking for: fried rice, fried shrimp, fried wontons, fried egg or spring rolls, fried calamari, tempura shrimp, and so on. Ask your server what kind of oil they use to prepare these items. Some restaurants use liquid sesame, soy, canola, or peanut oil instead of partially hydrogenated oil or shortening. If any of these items arrive at the restaurant already prepared, breaded, and/or precooked, they could very well contain partially hydrogenated oils, even though the cook may not use such oils to prepare them for you.

- Skip the fried noodles that are put on your table as an appetizer or with your meal.
- You can keep your saturated fat grams down, too, if you ask that your meal (vegetables, tofu, meats) be steamed or stir-fried with soy sauce instead of oil.
- If an entrée says "twice-cooked," it may mean the ingredients are fried after being boiled. Ask your server how the dish is prepared.

Mexican

- Tortilla chips and salsa are the trademarks of Mexican food. However, often the chips are made with partially hydrogenated oil. Ask your server to check the ingredients for you. Better yet, ask if you can have some warm tortillas instead of the chips. Just tear off a few pieces and dip into the salsa. Salsa is a great nonfat option instead of sour cream, guacamole, and cheese.
- Some fat-free ways to spice up your Mexican food include red chile sauce, ranchero sauce, tomatillo sauce (also known as green salsa or salsa verde), and pico de gallo (a hot relish).
- Since most Mexican food is made with some type of wrap or container (tortillas, taco shells), you need to ask about the ingredients in these items. Many commercially prepared taco shells and tortillas contain partially hydrogenated oils.

- Many Mexican food items are fried: refried beans, chimichangas, enchiladas, chalupas, sopapillas, even fried ice cream. In many places, restaurant owners have switched from lard (which has no trans fats but is high in saturated fat) to partially hydrogenated oil. Ask if your entrée can be baked instead of fried. Some restaurants may have nonrefried beans. Fajitas, burritos, quesadillas, tamales, and soft tacos typically are not fried.
- Instead of refried beans, ask if you can have charro or charra beans, which are seasoned pinto beans. Some restaurants make them fat free; others cook them with fat. Ask your server.

Indian/Middle Eastern

- Some Indian and Middle Eastern dishes are typically fried: for example, falafal, wheat gluten, poora (a popular type of pancake), bonda (fried vegetable fritter), pooris (deep-fried bread), bhatura (fried dough), and samosas (deep-fried stuffed pastry). Ask your server what type of oil is used for frying.
- Indian and Middle Eastern breads, pastries, and pancakes are traditionally made with liquid vegetable oil, not partially hydrogenated oils. Unless the cook prepares them using partially hydrogenated oil, they should be trans fat–free.
- Traditional Indian and Middle Eastern entrées make much use of lentils (especially in a popular dish called "dahl"), beans, vegetables, rice, pota-

toes, yogurt, chutney, and spices, which means you can feel quite sure about getting trans fat–free meals. When in doubt, always ask your server about ingredients.

Seafood

- Seafood is typically low in saturated fat, but if you order your fish breaded or batter-dipped and deep-fried, you've turned a potentially healthy meal into an artery-clogging one. Think broiled, grilled, steamed, or baked when ordering fish.
- Many seafood platters come with french fries, but you might want to order a baked potato instead and avoid the fat.

Vegetarian

- Vegetarian restaurants are more likely to, but will not always, use organic and/or whole foods (unprocessed), which means you probably won't have to worry about them serving foods that contain hydrogenated and partially hydrogenated oils. If you have any doubts, however, make sure to ask your server about ingredients.
- If you want to order a fried item, make sure you ask what type of oil they use.
- Just because a food is vegetarian doesn't mean it's automatically trans fat–free. If you batter-dip and deep-fry a perfectly healthy fresh vegetable or tofu in partially hydrogenated oil, you turn it

into a fatty food. Regular french fries are vegetarian (as long as they don't contain or aren't cooked in beef fat), but they may be deep-fried in partially hydrogenated oil.

GENERAL TIPS FOR EATING OUT

- If you eat at a fast-food restaurant, go in prepared. Read through the items in the lists provided in this book and identify those that are "best bets." When choosing your meal items, keep in mind your total recommended intake of total, saturated, and trans fats for the day. It's not hard to meet or surpass that amount for any of these categories when you eat just one fast-food sandwich or salad.
- Before you break bread, think. You may want to say no to the bread, crackers, chips, rolls, and bread sticks many restaurants put on your table, unless the management can guarantee their products don't contain trans fats.
- Look before you leap into the frying pan. If the food is fried in hydrogenated or partially hydrogenated oil, avoid it. Foods cooked in liquid vegetable oil may be trans fat–free, but their saturated fat levels are increased to varying degrees because of the oil, depending on which oil is used (see chart in chapter 2, "Breakdown of Fats in Different Oils"). Remember: Consider your trans and saturated fat quota for the day before you order. Depending on

the item, ask for it to be baked, broiled, steamed, or poached instead of fried. You may also ask if the item can be prepared in one of these ways, and then lightly sautéed in oil; or you can drizzle some healthy olive oil on the unfried food when it's brought to your table.

- Keep your salads healthy. Stay away from the fatty dressings, croutons, and crunchy Chinese noodles. Ask for olive oil or flaxseed oil and vinegar, lemon, salsa, garlic, herbs, or bring your own dressing from home.

- Request that your vegetables be prepared without oil or margarine. Besides, lightly steamed vegetables retain more of their nutritional value. Drizzle some olive oil or flaxseed oil on them for added flavor.

- Baked desserts—pies, cakes, cookies, brownies— as well as many puddings typically contain shortening or partially hydrogenated oils. To satisfy your sweet tooth, try fruit, sorbets, or low-fat frozen yogurt.

CHAPTER 5

Shopping for Your Family

Now that you know how to decipher Nutrition Facts panels and ingredient lists, you're ready to do some informed shopping. In this chapter we'll take you aisle by aisle through a virtual supermarket and look at the amount of total fat, saturated fat, and, when provided by the manufacturer, trans fats, in hundreds of food items. When manufacturers haven't provided the amount of trans fats, don't worry: You've already learned how to get a good idea of how much is in each product by reading the labels. Besides, we've provided you with a key so you know whether an item has a lot of trans fats, some trans fats, or no trans fats. At the end of each "aisle," we offer you a Best Bets list of trans fat–free—and low in saturated fat—alternatives for each category.

The foods listed here are only a sampling of the more than 320,000 items available on supermarket shelves. Because thousands of new products are introduced to the market every year (in 1998, for example, more than 11,000 new items were brought to market;

naturally, most don't succeed and are removed from the shelves), it's not possible to keep up with the large, rapid turnover of products. Thus we have mainly selected items that are popular, well-known, and/or are old standards (e.g., Kellogg's Corn Flakes, Campbell's Soup, Betty Crocker, Spam), plus some newer items that may have staying power. Fresh items (fruits, vegetables, meats, poultry, fish) are also included. It's possible you will see some items on the list that are not available in your area or in your markets. However, we trust the vast majority of foods will be familiar to you.

That being said, we want to emphasize that **trans fats are found in processed foods; the best way to avoid trans fats is to eliminate or significantly reduce the amount of processed foods in your diet and choose healthier, whole foods,** such as whole-grain breads, pastas, cereals, crackers, and snack foods; legumes, beans, fruits, vegetables, low-fat dairy products; fish, lean meats and poultry (organic preferred); and healthy oils, such as olive, flaxseed, and canola (remember—not all fats are bad!). Many of these items are available in mainstream supermarkets either in a natural foods section or next to conventional food items; you will find an even wider variety in natural and health food stores, food cooperatives, and farmers' markets. You will see some of these healthier choices listed on our food list.

We suggest you take this book with you while you shop and use it as a guide as you go up and down each aisle. So now, let's get ready to shop!

THE LABELS, THEY ARE A'CHANGIN'

As this book was being written, food manufacturers were gearing up to make labeling changes to their products. For some, the changes mean nothing more than adding "0 g trans fat" to their Nutrition Facts panels, because their products do not contain hydrogenated or partially hydrogenated oils. For others, it means identifying the amount of trans fats in their items and then taking one of two steps: listing the current amount on the label, or revamping their production process to reduce or eliminate these oils.

Some manufacturers decided to "beat the rush" and made product changes even before the Food and Drug Administration announced its ruling. Frito-Lay, for example, eliminated trans fats from nearly 90 percent of its products, including its corn chips, Cheetos, Tostitos, and Baked Doritos. Kraft Foods announced it was going to make some of its foods more heart-friendly by reducing fats, sugar, and calories.

Thus, labels and ingredient lists are changing and will continue to do so until January 2006, and probably beyond that time, as some food producers decide to make more ingredient changes based on consumer response and studies on the impact of certain ingredients on health. Therefore, you may notice that the fat gram figures for some products listed in this book will not match any new labeling that occurred after the writing of this book. This is an opportunity for you to make notations in the book for those products. In that way, you'll have the most up-to-date figures at your finger-tips whenever you shop.

After a few shopping trips, you will likely have identified most of the brands that fit your nutritional needs. We suggest, however, that you frequently check the Nutritional Facts panel and ingredient list for products you eat regularly. Manufacturers often make ingredient changes to their products, and you may not be aware of them. Hopefully, any changes will be for the better. To be sure, review labeling information every few months, especially if:

- the manufacturer has made color or size changes to the package and/or label;
- the manufacturer has added new wording such as "new," "improved," "now lower in fat," or similar claims.

HOW TO USE THE FOOD LISTS

The following food lists provide information about fat content per serving as defined on each item's packaging and, in some cases, based on the prepared product when made according to package directions. Note that foods shown as being low in fat are not necessarily healthy; they may contain high amounts of sugar, salt, white flour, chemical additives and preservatives, and/or be deficient in any number of essential nutrients. Information on cholesterol, sodium, total carbohydrates (fiber and sugars), protein, vitamins A and C, calcium, and iron are not provided in these lists; thus if you are interested in this information you are urged to read labels carefully. You are encouraged to eat a variety of foods throughout the day, including at least five servings of fruits and vegetables and 25 to 30 grams of fiber (found in whole grains, beans, legumes, fruits, and vegetables).

In the food lists, there are three columns to the right of each food item: "Total" (total fat), "Sat." (saturated fat), and "Trans" (trans fats). As we explained in earlier chapters, knowing the amounts of all three of these fats is important for your health, but especially trans fats, which we have focused on throughout this book. Although we have already shown you how you can, on your own, evaluate the amount of trans fats in products by looking at the ingredient panels, the following food lists, with the three columns, does the work for you. The "Total" fat column lets you know how much saturated, monounsaturated, polyunsaturated, and trans fats are in the item; the "Sat." column singles out the amount of harmful saturated fat; and the "Trans" column indicates whether the product has a high, medium to low, or no amount of hydrogenated or partially hydrogenated oil, shortening, or margarine, which are the indicators of the presence of trans fats. For optimum health for yourself and your family, you should keep track of your fat intake in these three categories and stay within the recommended limits, as shown in chapter 3.

At the end of each subsection in the lists is a heading called Best Bets. These items have no trans fats (no hydrogenated or partially hydrogenated oils or shortening) are low in saturated fat, with 2 grams or less (remember, you should watch your intake of trans fats plus saturated fat, as explained in chapter 3); and are low in total fat, with 4 grams or less (you want to keep your total fat intake to 30 percent or less of your total daily calories). When there are many Best Bets, we list the "best of the best"—those with no trans fats and the lowest saturated and total fat in the list. When there are no Best Bets in a section, we offer healthier alternatives, such as a similar but more nutritious item or a recipe or two from chapter 6.

KEY: Prepared = item prepared according to package directions. In some cases, you may be able to significantly reduce the amount of fat (trans and/or saturated fats) in the prepared item by eliminating or substituting one or more of the ingredients you are supposed to add to the recipe. Not Prepared = amounts shown are for the mix only, without the ingredients you need to add to complete the preparation. Addition of these ingredients may add a significant amount of saturated and/or trans fats to the final product. In the "Trans" column, "+" means hydrogenated or partially hydrogenated oil, shortening, or margarine is high on the list of ingredients; "–" means it is medium to low on the list; and "0" means it contains none of these ingredients.

BABY FOOD

Food Item	Total Fat	Sat. Fat	Trans Fat
Beech-Nut Table Time, Chicken & Stars	6	1.5	0
Beech-Nut Table Time, Macaroni & Cheese	7	4	0
Beech-Nut Table Time, Spaghetti Rings	6	4	0
Gerber Graduates, Beef & Tomato Ravioli	1.5	0.5	0
Gerber Graduates, Cheese Ravioli	3	1.5	-
Gerber Graduates, Chicken & Broccoli	5	3	0
Gerber Graduates, Macaroni & Beef	4	2	0
Gerber Graduates, Pasta Shells & Cheese	5	3.5	-
Gerber Graduates, Potatoes & Ham	5	3	-
Gerber Graduates, Spaghetti w/Meatballs	4	2	0
Gerber Graduates, Vegetable Stew w/Beef	2.5	1	0
Gerber Graduates, White Turkey Stew	3	1.5	0
Gerber Graduates Lil' Entrées, Chicken Noodle w/Oatmeal, Pears & Cinnamon	3	0	0
Gerber Graduates Lil' Entrées, Chicken Stew w/Noodles & Green Beans	3.5	1.5	0
Gerber Graduates Lil' Entrées, Pasta Wheels & Chicken w/Carrots	2	1	0

BABY FOOD *(cont.)*

Food Item	Total Fat	Sat. Fat	Trans Fat
Gerber Graduates for Toddlers, Apple Cinnamon Fruit & Cereal Bars	1.5	0	-
Gerber Graduates for Toddlers, Apple Graham Crisps	1	0	-
Gerber Graduates for Toddlers, Arrowroot Cookies	1	0	-
Gerber Graduates for Toddlers, Banana Cereal Snackin' Squares	1	0	0
Gerber Graduates for Toddlers, Veggie Crackers	1.5	0	+

BEST BETS: All foods contain acceptable ranges of fat for infants and toddlers.

BAKED GOODS

Food Item	Total Fat	Sat. Fat	Trans Fat
Bagels/English Muffins			
Burns & Ricker Bagel Crisps, Cinnamon Raisin	5	1	+
Burns & Ricker Bagel Crisps, Everything	6	1	+
Burns & Ricker Bagel Crisps, Plain	4.5	0.5	+
Oroweat Australian Toaster Biscuits	6	1.5	+
Oroweat English Muffins, Extra Crisp	1	0	-
Oroweat English Muffins, Health Nut	3	0	0

BAKED GOODS *(cont.)*

Food Item	Total Fat	Sat. Fat	Trans Fat
Oroweat English Muffins, Sourdough	1	0	-
Sara Lee Bagels, Banana Walnut	7	2.5	0
Sara Lee Bagels, Blueberry	1	0	0
Sara Lee Bagels, Cinnamon Raisin	1	0	0
Sara Lee Bagels, Cranberry Orange	1.5	0	0
Sara Lee Bagels, Plain or Onion	1	0	0
Sara Lee Bagels, Sun Dried Tomato & Basil	1.5	0	0
Thomas' Bagels, 100% Whole Wheat	2	1	0
Thomas' Bagels, Blueberry	2	0.5	-
Thomas' Bagels, Cinnamon Raisin Swirl	2	0.5	0
Thomas' Bagels, Everything	4	1	0
Thomas' English Muffins, Original	1	0	0
Thomas' English Muffins, Cinnamon Raisin	1	0	-
Thomas' English Muffins, Sourdough	1	0	0

BEST BETS: Oroweat English Muffins, Health Nut; Sara Lee Bagels, all except Banana Walnut; Thomas' Bagels, all except Blueberry; Thomas' English Muffins, Original and Sourdough

Bread/Rolls

Aunt Hattie's Homestyle w/Buttermilk	1.5	0	-
Aunt Hattie's Homestyle Light 9 Grain	1	0	0

THE TRANS FAT REMEDY

BAKED GOODS *(cont.)*

Food Item	Total Fat	Sat. Fat	Trans Fat
Aunt Hattie's Homestyle Potato	1	0	-
Aunt Hattie's Homestyle Wheat	1.5	0	-
Earth Grains Honey Wheat Berry Buns	2.5	0.5	0
Earth Grains Onion Buns	2	0.5	0
Earth Grains Soft Hoagies	3	0.5	-
IronKids Bread, No Crust	1	0	0
IronKids Bread, Wheat	0.5	0	0
King's Hawaiian Sweet Bread	4.5	1.5	+
King's Hawaiian Sweet Rolls	2	1	+
King's Hawaiian Sweet Rolls, Sandwich	6	2	+
Oroweat 100% Whole Wheat	1	0	0
Oroweat Cinnamon Swirl	3	0.5	-
Oroweat Country Potato	1	0	-
Oroweat Country Rye	1.5	0	-
Oroweat Dark Rye	1	0	0
Oroweat Dark Wheat	1.5	0	-
Oroweat Extra Sour Rye	1	0	-
Oroweat Healthy Multi-Grain	1.5	0	0
Oroweat Milk & Honey	1.5	0	-
Oroweat Oatnut	2	0.5	-
Oroweat Raisin Bread Cinnamon Swirl	1	0	-
Pepperidge Farm 9 Grain	1.5	0	0
Pepperidge Farm German Dark Wheat	1.5	0	0
Pepperidge Farm, Farmhouse Crunchy Oat	1.5	0	0

BAKED GOODS *(cont.)*

Food Item	Total Fat	Sat. Fat	Trans Fat
Pepperidge Farm, Farmhouse Harvest 7 Grain	1	0	0
Pepperidge Farm, Farmhouse Hearty White	1	0	0
Pepperidge Farm, Farmhouse Sweet Buttermilk	1	0	-
Sara Lee 100% Whole Wheat	1.5	0	0
Sara Lee Honey White	0.5	0	0
Sara Lee 6 Grain	0.5	0	0
Sun-Maid Raisin Bread, Cinnamon Swirl	1.5	0.5	-
Wonder Light, Low Fat	0.5	0	0
Wonder Light, Wheat	0.5	0	0
Wonder Large White	1	0	0
Wonder Thin Sandwich	1	0	0

BEST BETS: Aunt Hattie's 9 Grain; IronKids Bread; Oroweat 100% Wheat and Oroweat Healthy Multi-Grain; Pepperidge Farm, all except Sweet Buttermilk; Sara Lee, all; Wonder, all

Cakes/Snack Cakes

Food Item	Total Fat	Sat. Fat	Trans Fat
Entenmann's Banana Cake	15	3.5	+
Entenmann's Cheese Filled Crumb Coffee Cake	10	3	-
Entenmann's Cheese Topped Coffee Cake	9	2.5	-
Entenmann's Cinnamon Swirl Buns	14	3.5	+
Entenmann's Golden Loaf, Fat Free	0	0	0

BAKED GOODS *(cont.)*

Food Item	Total Fat	Sat. Fat	Trans Fat
Entenmann's Lemon Crunch Cake	13	3.5	+
Entenmann's Louisiana Crunch Cake	15	4	+
Entenmann's Marshmallow Iced Devil's Food Cake	14	3.5	+
Entenmann's New York Crumb Coffee Cake	12	3	+
Entenmann's Light Raspberry Twist Danish	0	0	0
Hostess Brownie Bites	9	2	+
Hostess Cinnamon Streusel Cakes	6	2	+
Hostess Ding Dongs	19	2	+
Hostess Golden Cupcakes	7	3	+
Hostess Ho Hos	12	8	+
Hostess Mini Muffins, Blueberry	8	1	+
Hostess Pies, Apple	22	9	+
Hostess Pies, Blackberry	21	11	+
Hostess Pies, Cherry	22	11	+
Hostess Pies, Lemon	24	11	+
Hostess SnoBalls	5	2.5	+
Hostess Twinkies	5	2	+
Little Debbie Chocolate Chip Cakes	15	3.5	+
Little Debbie Coffee Cakes, Apple Streusel	7	1.5	+
Little Debbie Devil Squares	13	3	+
Little Debbie Donut Sticks	14	3.5	+
Little Debbie Fancy Cakes	15	3.5	+
Little Debbie Fudge Rounds	6	1.5	+
Little Debbie Golden Cremes	4.5	1.5	-

BAKED GOODS *(cont.)*

Food Item	Total Fat	Sat. Fat	Trans Fat
Little Debbie Honey Buns	13	3.5	+
Little Debbie Nutty Bars	18	4	+
Little Debbie Oatmeal Creme Pies	7	1.5	+
Little Debbie Pecan Spinwheels	4	0.5	-
Little Debbie Star Crunch	6	1.5	+
Little Debbie Strawberry Shortcake Rolls	8	2	+
Little Debbie Swirl Cake Rolls	12	3	+
Little Debbie Zebra Cakes	16	3.5	+
Otis Spunkmeyer Breakfast Claws	12	3.5	+
Otis Spunkmeyer Fruit Danish	12	3	+
Otis Spunkmeyer Muffins, Banana Nut	12	2	0
Otis Spunkmeyer Muffins, Chocolate Chocolate Chip	12	2.5	0
Otis Spunkmeyer Muffins, Wild Blueberry	11	2.5	0

BEST BETS: Entenmann's Fat-Free Golden Loaf and Light Raspberry Twist Danish

Doughnuts

	Total Fat	Sat. Fat	Trans Fat
Entenmann's Frosted Devil's Food Popems	15	4	+
Entenmann's Glazed Buttermilk Donuts	13	3	+
Entenmann's Glazed Popems	12	3	+

BAKED GOODS (cont.)

Food Item	Total Fat	Sat. Fat	Trans Fat
Entenmann's Milk Chocolatey Donuts	19	5	+
Entenmann's Rich Frosted Devil's Food Donuts	19	5	+
Hostess Crumb Donettes	10	4.5	+
Hostess Frosted Donettes	14	8	+
Krispy Kreme Glazed Doughnuts	12	3	+

BEST BETS: None, unless you can find a fat-free variety. Instead of a doughnut, try a whole-grain bagel or English muffin with whole fruit jam or honey.

Pizza Crusts

Boboli Mini Crusts	3	0.5	0
Boboli Original Pizza Crust	2.5	0	+
Boboli Thin Pizza Crust	3.5	0.5	+

BEST BET: Boboli Mini Crusts

Stuffing

Butterball Stuffing (box), Chicken, not prepared	3.5	0	0
Butterball Stuffing (box), Seasoned, not prepared	3.5	0	0
Mrs. Cubbison's Herb Seasoning, not prepared	1.5	0	-
Mrs. Cubbison's Seasoned, not prepared	1	0	-
Mrs. Cubbison's Seasoned Cornbread, not prepared	1	0	-

BAKED GOODS *(cont.)*

Food Item	Total Fat	Sat. Fat	Trans Fat
Stove Top Stuffing, Cornbread, prepared	8	1.5	-
Stove Top Stuffing, Pork, prepared	9	2	-
Stove Top Stuffing, Chicken, prepared	9	2	-
Stove Top Stuffing, Mushroom & Onion, prepared	9	2	-
Stove Top Stuffing, Savory Herb, prepared	9	2	-

BEST BETS: Mrs. Cubbison's varieties, but don't use partially hydrogenated shortening to prepare them.

Tacos/Tortillas

Food Item	Total Fat	Sat. Fat	Trans Fat
Arizona Corn Tortillas	1	0	0
Arizona Flour Tortillas, premium jumbo	5	1.5	+
Arizona Flour Tortillas, Low Fat, burrito size	2	0	-
Arizona Whole Wheat Tortillas	3.5	1	+
Casa Fiesta Taco Shells	6	5	+
Mission Corn Tortillas, white, small	2	0.5	0
Mission Corn Tortillas, yellow, super size	1	0.5	0
Mission Flour Tortillas, burrito size	0.5	0	-
Mission Flour Tortillas, fajita size	3	0.5	+
Mission Flour Tortillas, soft taco size	3	1	+

BAKED GOODS (cont.)

Food Item	Total Fat	Sat. Fat	Trans Fat
Mission Whole Wheat Tortillas, 96% Fat Free	2.5	0.5	-
Old El Paso Taco Shells, white corn	7	2	+
Ortega Taco Shells, yellow corn	5	1	+
Rosarita Taco Shells	4	1	+

BEST BETS: All corn and flour tortillas (except premium jumbo Arizona Flour Tortillas). Avoid taco shells.

BAKING INGREDIENTS

Note: Amounts listed for mixes refer to the mix only, not the prepared product. Remember that adding ingredients will likely change the amount of total, saturated, and/or trans fats in the finished product.

Food Item	Total Fat	Sat. Fat	Trans Fat
Basic Mixes			
Bisquick	6	1.5	+
Bisquick, Reduced Fat	3	0.5	+
Jiffy Baking Mix	4.5	1	+

BEST BETS: None. Try the Anytime Biscuits recipe in chapter 6.

Cake Mixes			
Banquet Dessert Bakes, Apple Crisp	3.5	0.5	+
Banquet Dessert Bakes, Cherry Cobbler	4	1	+
Banquet Dessert Bakes, Peach Cobbler	4	1	+

BAKING INGREDIENTS *(cont.)*

Food Item	Total Fat	Sat. Fat	Trans Fat
Banquet Dessert Bakes, Chocolate Cherry Decadence	5	2	+
Banquet Dessert Bakes, Chocolate Lava Cake	7	1.5	+
Betty Crocker Gingerbread Cake Mix	6	1.5	+
Betty Crocker Pound Cake Mix	7	2.5	+
Betty Crocker Complete Desserts, Apple Crisp	6	1.5	+
Betty Crocker Complete Desserts, Cherry Cobbler	7	2	+
Betty Crocker Complete Desserts, Peach Cobbler	7	1.5	+
Betty Crocker Snackin' Cakes, Cinnamon Swirl	5	1.5	+
Betty Crocker Snackin' Cakes, German Chocolate	5	2.5	+
Betty Crocker Super Moist, Carrot Cake	3	1	+
Betty Crocker Super Moist, Devil's Food Cake	2.5	1	+
Betty Crocker Super Moist, French Vanilla	3	1.5	+
Betty Crocker Super Moist, Fudge Marble	4	1.5	+
Betty Crocker Super Moist, German Chocolate	2.5	1	+
Betty Crocker Super Moist, Triple Chocolate Fudge	4	2	+

BAKING INGREDIENTS *(cont.)*

Food Item	Total Fat	Sat. Fat	Trans Fat
Duncan Hines Angel Food, fat free	0	0	0
Duncan Hines Butter Recipe, Golden	5	2	+
Duncan Hines Classic Yellow	3	1	+
Duncan Hines Devil's Food	3.5	1.5	+
Duncan Hines Lemon Supreme	4	1.5	+
Duncan Hines Pineapple Supreme	4	1.5	+
Duncan Hines Spice	4	1.5	+
Krusteaz Cinnamon Crumb Cake	7	2	+
Pillsbury Moist Supreme, Butter Recipe	3	1	+
Pillsbury Moist Supreme, Fudge Swirl	2.5	1	+
Pillsbury Moist Supreme, Funetti	4	1.5	+
Pillsbury Moist Supreme, German Chocolate	4	1.5	+
Pillsbury Moist Supreme, White	4	1.5	+

BEST BET: Duncan Hines Angel Food

Cookie/Brownie Mixes

Food Item	Total Fat	Sat. Fat	Trans Fat
Betty Crocker Brownie, Original Supreme	1.5	0.5	+
Betty Crocker Brownie, Triple Chunk	3	1.5	+
Betty Crocker Brownie, Walnut Chocolate Chunk	3.5	1	+
Betty Crocker Oatmeal Cookie Mix	1.5	0	-
Betty Crocker Oatmeal Chocolate Chip Cookie Mix	3	1	-
Betty Crocker Peanut Butter Cookie Mix	3.5	0.5	+

BAKING INGREDIENTS *(cont.)*

Food Item	Total Fat	Sat. Fat	Trans Fat
Betty Crocker Rainbow Chocolate Candy Cookie Mix	2	1	-
Betty Crocker Sugar Cookie Mix	3	0.5	+
Duncan Hines Brownies, Candy Shop M&M's	2.5	1	+
Duncan Hines Brownies, Candy Shop Twix	3	1	+
Krusteaz Key Lime Bar Mix	3	0	+
Krusteaz Lemon Bar Mix	3	0	+
Pillsbury Rich & Moist Brownies	2.5	0.5	+
Pillsbury Thick 'N Fudgy Cheesecake Swirl Brownie	3	1	+
Pillsbury Thick 'N Fudgy Deluxe Brownie, Walnut	4.5	1	+
Pillsbury Thick 'N Fudgy Vanilla Frosted	3.5	1	+

BEST BET: Betty Crocker Oatmeal Cookie Mix; also try the Brownie recipe in chapter 6.

Chips

Baker's German Sweet Chocolate Bar	3.5	2	0
Baker's Unsweetened Chocolate Baking Bar	7	4.5	0
Hershey's Milk Chocolate Chips	4.5	2.5	0
Hershey's Semi-Sweet Chips	4.5	2.5	0
Hershey's Unsweetened Chocolate Baking Bar	7	4.5	0

BAKING INGREDIENTS *(cont.)*

Food Item	Total Fat	Sat. Fat	Trans Fat
Nestlé Butterscotch Chips	4	3.5	+
Nestlé Chocolate Chunk	3.5	2	0
Nestlé Milk Chocolate Morsels	4.5	2.5	0
Nestlé Peanut Butter and Milk Chocolate Morsels	4.5	3	-
Nestlé Premier White Morsels	4	3.5	-
Nestlé Semi-Sweet Morsels	4	2.5	0
Reese's Peanut Butter Chips	4	4	+
Reese's Peanut Butter and Milk Chocolate Chips	4.5	3	-
Skor English Toffee Bits	4.5	2.5	0

BEST BETS: Baker's German Sweet Chocolate bar; Nestlé Chocolate Chunk. Both are high in sugar, however, and thus not a nutritional "best bet."

Frostings

	Total Fat	Sat. Fat	Trans Fat
Betty Crocker, Caramel	5	1.5	+
Betty Crocker, Chocolate Almond	8	3	+
Betty Crocker, Coconut Pecan	8	3	+
Betty Crocker, Cream Cheese	8	3	+
Betty Crocker, Lemon	8	3	+
Betty Crocker, Milk Chocolate	5	1.5	+
Betty Crocker, Whipped Chocolate	5	1.5	+
Betty Crocker, Whipped Fluffy White	4.5	1.5	+
Betty Crocker, Whipped Vanilla	6	1	+
Duncan Hines Creamy Home Style Frosting, Classic Chocolate	5	1.5	+

BAKING INGREDIENTS *(cont.)*

Food Item	Total Fat	Sat. Fat	Trans Fat
Duncan Hines Creamy Home Style Frosting, Classic Vanilla	5	1.5	+
Duncan Hines Creamy Home Style Frosting, Cream Cheese	5	1.5	+
Duncan Hines Creamy Home Style Frosting, Fun Frosters	6	1.5	+
Duncan Hines Creamy Home Style Frosting, Milk Chocolate	5	1.5	+
Duncan Hines Creamy Home Style Frosting, White Chocolate Almond	5	1.5	+
Pillsbury Creamy Supreme, Chocolate Walnut	7	1.5	+
Pillsbury Creamy Supreme, Coconut Pecan	10	4	+
Pillsbury Creamy Supreme, Confetti Funfetti	6	1.5	+
Pillsbury Creamy Supreme, Cream Cheese	6	1.5	+
Pillsbury Creamy Supreme, Milk Chocolate	6	1.5	+
Pillsbury Creamy Supreme, Vanilla	6	1.5	+
Pillsbury Creamy Supreme, Vanilla Almond	6	1.5	+

BEST BETS: None. Try topping your cakes and cupcakes with pureed fruit and chopped nuts or whipped low-fat cream cheese and raisins.

BAKING INGREDIENTS *(cont.)*

Food Item	Total Fat	Sat. Fat	Trans Fat
Muffin/Quick Bread Mixes			
Betty Crocker Banana Nut Muffin Mix	3	0.5	-
Betty Crocker Banana Quick Bread Mix	2.5	0.5	+
Betty Crocker Cinnamon Streusel Muffin Mix	4	1	+
Betty Crocker Cinnamon Streusel Quick Bread Mix	4.5	1	+
Betty Crocker Lemon Poppy Seed Quick Bread Mix	2.5	0.5	+
Betty Crocker Wild Blueberry Muffin Mix	1.5	0	-
Duncan Hines Blueberry Streusel Muffins	4.5	1	+
Krusteaz Apple Cinnamon Muffins; also Cranberry Orange, Wild Blueberry; all Fat Free	0	0	0
Krusteaz Oat Bran Muffin Mix	4	1	+
Krusteaz Wild Blueberry Muffin Mix	4	1	+
Pillsbury Carrot Cake Muffin Mix	4	1	+
Pillsbury Chocolate Chip Muffin Mix	6	2	+

BEST BETS: Krusteaz Fat-Free mixes, all

Pancake/Waffle Mixes			
Aunt Jemima Buttermilk Complete	2.5	0.5	-
Aunt Jemima Complete	2	0.5	-
Krusteaz Belgian Waffle Mix	2.5	0.5	-
Krusteaz Blueberry Pancake Mix	3	0.5	-

BAKING INGREDIENTS (cont.)

Food Item	Total Fat	Sat. Fat	Trans Fat
Krusteaz Buttermilk Pancake Mix	2.5	0.5	-
Krusteaz Wheat & Honey Pancake Mix	1.5	0.5	0

BEST BET: Krusteaz Wheat & Honey pancake mix; also try the Apple Waffle recipe in chapter 6.

Pie Crusts

Keebler, Chocolate	5	1	+
Keebler, Graham Cracker	6	1.5	+
Keebler, Shortbread	5	1	+
Nabisco, Honey Maid	8	1.5	+
Nabisco, Nilla	8	1.5	+
Nabisco, Oreo	7	1.5	+

BEST BETS: None. Try the low-fat pie crust recipe (see Blueberry Pie) in chapter 6.

Pie Fillings

Comstock Pie Filling, Red Ruby Cherry	0	0	0
Comstock Pie Filling, More Fruit, all flavors	0	0	0
Libby's Pumpkin	0.5	0	0
Solo Almond Filling	2.5	0.5	0
Solo Poppy Seed Filling	4	0	0
Solo Prune Plum Filling	0	0	0
Solo Strawberry Filling	0	0	0

BEST BETS: all

BAKING INGREDIENTS *(cont.)*

Food Item	Total Fat	Sat. Fat	Trans Fat
Pudding Cups			
Hunt's Snack Pack, Banana Cream Pie	6	1.5	+
Hunt's Snack Pack, Chocolate Boo	5	1.5	+
Hunt's Snack Pack, Chocolate Fudge	5	1.5	+
Hunt's Snack Pack, Chocolate Mud Pie	7	2	+
Hunt's Snack Pack, Cookies & Scream	4.5	1.5	+
Hunt's Snack Pack, Lemon Meringue	3	1	+
Hunt's Snack Pack, Strawberry Pow	4.5	1.5	+
Hunt's Snack Pack, Tapioca	4.5	1	+
Hunt's Snack Pack, Vanilla	4.5	1.5	+
Hunt's Squeeze 'n Go Pudding Tube, Chocolate	3	1	+
Kraft Handi-Snacks, Banana Pudding	4	1	+
Kraft Handi-Snacks, Butterscotch Pudding	3.5	1	+
Kraft Handi-Snacks, Chocolate Pudding	3.5	1	+
Kraft Handi-Snacks, Fat Free, all flavors	0	0	0
Kraft Handi-Snacks, Rice Pudding	6	1	+
Kraft Handi-Snacks, Vanilla Pudding	3.5	1	+

BEST BETS: Kraft Handi-Snacks, Fat Free, all flavors. Also try the Chocolate Pudding recipe in chapter 6.

BEVERAGES

Note: Alcoholic beverages, soda, flavored waters, bottled (nonfrozen or unrefrigerated) fruit and vegetable juices, and unprocessed teas and coffees are fat free, so we have not listed them here. This aisle is reserved for a variety of other beverages that contain fat, including flavored coffees and hot cocoa mixes and diet/supplement drinks.

Food Item	Total Fat	Sat. Fat	Trans Fat
Diet/Supplement Drinks			
EAS Advant Edge Shakes, Chocolate Fudge	3	0.5	0
EAS Advant Edge Shakes, French Vanilla	4	0	0
EAS Advant Edge Shakes, Strawberry Banana Twist	3	0	0
Ensure Butter Pecan Drink	6	0.5	0
Ensure Chocolate Drink	6	0.5	0
Ensure Chocolate Royale Drink	6	0.5	0
Ensure Coffee Latte Drink	6	0.5	0
Ensure Wild Berry Drink	6	0.5	0
Slim-Fast Meal Options, French Vanilla, can	2.5	0.5	0
Slim-Fast Meal Options, Orange-Strawberry-Banana	1	0	0
Slim-Fast Meal Options, Strawberry 'N Cream	2.5	0.5	0
Slim-Fast Soy Protein Meal Option, Café Mocha	1.5	0.5	0
Slim-Fast Soy Protein Meal Option, Chocolate Delite	2	1	0

BEST BETS: All except Ensure.

BEVERAGES *(cont.)*

Food Item	Total Fat	Sat. Fat	Trans Fat
Flavored Coffees			
Folgers Café Latte, Caramel Groove	5	2	+
Folgers Café Latte, Mocha Fusion	5	2	+
Folgers Café Latte, Vanilla Vibe	5	2	+
General Foods Intl. Coffee, Café Francais	3.5	1	+
General Foods Intl. Coffee, French Vanilla Café, fat free	0	0	-
General Foods Intl. Coffee, International Cappuccino	2.5	0.5	+
General Foods Intl. Coffee, Kahlua Café	2	0.5	+
General Foods Intl. Coffee, Orange Cappuccino	2	0.5	+
General Foods Intl. Coffee, Suisse Mocha	2	0.5	+
General Foods Intl. Coffee, Swiss White Chocolate	3	0.5	+
General Foods Intl. Coffee, Viennese Chocolate Café	1.5	0.5	+
Nescafé Frothé, Butterfinger	3	2	+
Nescafé Frothé, Captivating Caramel	3	2	+
Nescafé Frothé, Divinely Mocha	3	2	+
Nescafé Frothé, Enchanting Vanilla	3	2	+
Nescafé Frothé, Mystical Hazelnut Mocha	3	2	+
Nescafé Frothé, Silky White Chocolate	3	2	+

BEST BETS: None. Make your own coffee and add a flavored nonfat, nondairy creamer (see Creamers under the "Dairy" heading).

BEVERAGES *(cont.)*

Food Item	Total Fat	Sat. Fat	Trans Fat
Hot Cocoa/Malt Mixes			
Nestlé Hot Cocoa, Butterfinger	3	2	+
Nestlé Hot Cocoa, Milk Chocolate	2.5	1.5	+
Nestlé Hot Cocoa w/Mini Marshmallows	3	2	+
Nestlé Nesquik Hot Cocoa	3	2.5	+
Nestlé Hot Cocoa, Rich Chocolate	3	2	+
Ovaltine Chocolate Malt	0	0	0
Ovaltine Malt	0	0	0
Ovaltine Rich Chocolate	0	0	0
Swiss Miss Milk Chocolate	2.5	1	+
Swiss Miss Milk Chocolate w/Marshmallows	2.5	0.5	+
Swiss Miss No Sugar Added, w/Calcium	1	0	+

BEST BETS: Ovaltine, all

CANDY & DESSERT TOPPINGS

Note: Serving sizes of candy bars are given in grams, as candy tends to come in several different sizes, and manufacturers often change the size of their products. Read labels carefully.

Food Item	Total Fat	Sat. Fat	Trans Fat
Candy Bars			
Hershey's 5th Avenue, 33 grams	7	2.5	-
Hershey's Kisses	13	8	0
Hershey's KitKat, 42 grams	11	7	0
Hershey's Milk Chocolate, 43 grams	13	9	0

CANDY & DESSERT TOPPINGS *(cont.)*

Food Item	Total Fat	Sat. Fat	Trans Fat
Hershey's PayDay, 19 grams	5	4	0
M&M/Mars, Milky Way, 58.1 grams	10	5	-
M&M/Mars, M&M's, Original	9	6	0
M&M/Mars, M&M's, Peanut	12	6	-
M&M/Mars, Snickers, 58.7 grams	14	5	-
M&M/Mars, 3 Musketeers, 60.4 grams	8	4.5	-
M&M/Mars, Twix, 56.7 grams	14	5	-
Nestlé Baby Ruth, 60 grams	14	8	+
Nestlé Butterfinger, 60 grams	11	6	+
Nestlé Crunch, 44 grams	12	7	0
Peter Paul Almond Joy, 19 grams	5	3.5	-
Peter Paul Mounds, 19 grams	5	4	0
Reese's Peanut Butter Cup, 42 grams	13	5	0

BEST BETS: None. Satisfy your sweet tooth with fresh fruit, dried fruit like raisins or banana chips, or one of the candies listed under Other below.

Candy/Other

Hershey's KitKat Bites	10	7	-
Hershey's Milk Chocolate w/Almond Bites	14	7	-
Jelly Belly Jelly Beans	0	0	0
Jolly Rancher Hard Candy	0	0	0
Jolly Rancher Fruit Chews Lollipops	0	0	-
Kraft Creme Savers, Hard Candy, Chocolate & Caramel	1.5	1	-

CANDY & DESSERT TOPPINGS *(cont.)*

Food Item	Total Fat	Sat. Fat	Trans Fat
Kraft Creme Savers, Hard Candy, Chocolate & Caramel, sugar free	1.5	1	-
Kraft Creme Savers, Hard Candy, Orange	1.5	1.5	+
Kraft Creme Savers, Hard Candy, Peaches & Creme	1.5	1.5	+
Kraft Creme Savers, Soft Candy, Chocolate & Caramel	3.5	2.5	+
Kraft Creme Savers, Soft Candy, Orange & Creme	4	3	+
Kraft Creme Savers, Soft Candy, Strawberry & Creme	4	3.5	+
Nestlé Raisinets	8	5	0
Nestlé Signatures Treasures, Chocolate Creme	10	6	-
Nestlé Signatures Treasures, Creamy Caramel	9	5	-
Nestlé Signatures Treasures, Peanut Butter	13	7	+
Nestlé Signatures Treasures, Toasted Coconut	12	8	-
Peter Paul Almond Joy Bites	14	8	-
Reese's Bites	12	7	-
Skittles, Original	2	0	+
Skittles, Sour	1.5	0	+

CANDY & DESSERT TOPPINGS *(cont.)*

Food Item	Total Fat	Sat. Fat	Trans Fat
Starburst Fruit Chews, Original	3.5	0.5	+
Starburst Fruit Chews, Tropical	3	0.5	+
Starburst Jelly Beans	0	0	0
York Peppermint Bites	3	1.5	0

BEST BETS: Jelly Belly Jelly Beans, Jolly Rancher Hard Candy, Starburst Jelly Beans

Dessert Toppings

Food Item	Total Fat	Sat. Fat	Trans Fat
Hershey's Hot Cocoa Collection, Chocolate Raspberry	3	0.5	+
Hershey's Hot Cocoa Collection, Dutch Chocolate, Fat Free	0	0	0
Hershey's Hot Cocoa Collection, French Vanilla	2.5	0	+
Hershey's Hot Fudge Topping	5	2	-
Hershey's Shell, Chocolate	18	7	+
Hershey's Strawberry Syrup	0	0	0
Hershey's Syrup, can	0	0	0
Smucker's Magic Shell, Turtle Delight	16	7	+
Smucker's Magic Shell, Twix	15	7	+
Smucker's Milk Caramel Topping	4	1.5	+
Smucker's Sundae Syrup Caramel, Fat Free	0	0	0
Smucker's 3 Musketeers Sundae Syrup	2	1	-

CANDY & DESSERT TOPPINGS *(cont.)*

Food Item	Total Fat	Sat. Fat	Trans Fat
Smucker's Topping, Hot Fudge	4	1	-
Smucker's Topping, Milky Way	4	1.5	-

BEST BETS: Hershey's Dutch Chocolate, Fat Free; Hershey's Strawberry Syrup; Hershey's Syrup (can); Smucker's Sundae Syrup, Caramel Fat Free

CEREALS & CEREAL FOODS

Food Item	Total Fat	Sat. Fat	Trans Fat
Cereals, Cold			
General Mills Basic 4	3	0	-
General Mills Cheerios	2	0	0
General Mills Cheerios, Apple Cinnamon	1.5	0	-
General Mills Cheerios, Multigrain	1	0	-
General Mills Corn Chex	0	0	0
General Mills Count Chocula	1	0	-
General Mills Honey Nut Cheerios	1.5	0	0
General Mills Honey Nut Clusters	2.5	0	0
General Mills Lucky Charms	1	0	0
General Mills Raisin Nut Bran	4	0.5	0
General Mills Reese's Puffs	3	0.5	-
General Mills Total	1	0	0
General Mills Trix	1	0	-
General Mills Wheat Chex	1	0	0
General Mills Wheaties, frosted	0	0	0
Kashi GoLean Crunch	3	0	0
Kashi Good Friends, Cinna-Raisin Crunch	1.5	0	0

CEREALS & CEREAL FOODS *(cont.)*

Food Item	Total Fat	Sat. Fat	Trans Fat
Kashi Heart to Heart	1.5	0	0
Kashi Honey Puffed	1	0	0
Kashi Organic Promise, Strawberry Fields	0	0	0
Kashi Organic Promise, Cranberry Sunshine	1	0	0
Kashi, Puffed	0.5	0	0
Kellogg's Apple Jacks	0.5	0	-
Kellogg's Cocoa Krispies	1	0.5	-
Kellogg's Corn Pops	0	0	-
Kellogg's Frosted Mini-Wheats	1	0	0
Kellogg's Fruit Harvest, Strawberry or Blueberry	1.5	0	0
Kellogg's Froot Loops	1	0.5	-
Kellogg's Product 19	0	0	0
Kellogg's Raisin Bran	1.5	0	0
Kellogg's Rice Krispies	0	0	0
Kellogg's Smart Start	0.5	0	0
Kellogg's Smart Start, Soy Protein	1.5	0	0
Post Fruity Pebbles	1	1	+
Post Golden Crisp	1	0	-
Post Grape-Nuts	1	0	0
Post Grape-Nuts Flakes	1	0	-
Post Great Grains Select, Crunchy Pecans	6	1	+
Post Honey Bunches of Oats w/Strawberries	2	0	+
Post Honey Comb	0.5	0	0

CEREALS & CEREAL FOODS *(cont.)*

Food Item	Total Fat	Sat. Fat	Trans Fat
Post Shredded Wheat	1	0	0
Post Shredded Wheat, Honey Nut	1.5	0	-
Post Waffle Crisp	2.5	0	-
Quaker 100% Natural Granola, Oats, Honey & Raisin	8	3.5	-
Quaker 100% Natural Granola, low fat, w/raisins	3	1	-
Quaker Cap'n Crunch	1.5	0.5	-
Quaker Honey Graham Oh's	2	0.5	+
Quaker Life, Original	1.5	0	0
Quaker Life, Cinnamon	1.5	0	0
Quaker Oat Bran	3	0.5	0

BEST BETS: These are the best of the best: General Mills: Cheerios, Corn Chex, Honey Nut Cheerios, Total, Wheat Chex; Kashi: Heart to Heart, Honey Puffed, Organic Promise; Kellogg's: Fruit Harvest, Product 19, Raisin Bran, Rice Krispies, Smart Start, Smart Start Soy; Post: Grape-Nuts, Shredded Wheat; Quaker: Life, Original and Cinnamon. Many other cereals fit the criteria for "Best Bets," but because they contain much sugar, we did not list them. We suggest you read the ingredient lists for sugar content on cereals before you purchase them. If sugar is one of the first two or three ingredients, the product is best avoided. You can naturally sweeten nonsugary cereals with the herbal sweetener stevia, or use fresh fruit or raisins.

Food Item	Total Fat	Sat. Fat	Trans Fat
Cereals, Hot			
Nabisco Cream of Wheat, Instant, Maple Brown Sugar	0	0	0

CEREALS & CEREAL FOODS *(cont.)*

Food Item	Total Fat	Sat. Fat	Trans Fat
Nabisco Cream of Wheat, Original	0	0	0
Nabisco Cream of Wheat, Peaches & Cream	1.5	0	+
Nabisco Cream of Wheat, Strawberry & Cream	1.5	0	+
Quaker Instant Oatmeal, Baked Apple	2	0	0
Quaker Instant Oatmeal, Cinnamon & Spice	2	0.5	0
Quaker Instant Oatmeal, French Vanilla	2	0	0
Quaker Instant Oatmeal, Raisin Cinnamon Swirl	2	0.5	0
Quaker Instant Oatmeal, Raisin & Spice	2	0.5	0
Quaker Instant Oatmeal, Strawberry & Cream	2.5	0.5	+

BEST BETS: Nabisco Cream of Wheat, Instant, Maple Brown Sugar; Nabisco Cream of Wheat, Original; Quaker Instant Oatmeal, all except Strawberry & Cream

Breakfast Bars

Food Item	Total Fat	Sat. Fat	Trans Fat
General Mills Milk 'n Cereal Bars, Honey Nut Cheerios	4	1.5	+
General Mills Milk 'n Cereal Bars, Cocoa Puffs	4	1.5	+
General Mills Oatmeal Crisp Fruit 'n Cereal Bars, Apple Cinnamon	2	0	-

CEREALS & CEREAL FOODS (cont.)

Food Item	Total Fat	Sat. Fat	Trans Fat
General Mills Oatmeal Crisp Fruit 'n Cereal Bars, Blueberry; also Strawberry	2	0	-
Health Valley Cereal Bars, Apple Cobbler	2	0	0
Health Valley Cereal Bars, Blueberry; also Fig and Strawberry	2	0	0
Health Valley Granola Bars, Chocolate Chip, Date-Almond Raspberry, Fat Free	0	0	0
Health Valley Tarts, Blueberry, Chocolate, Red Cherry	2	0	0
Kellogg's Cereal & Milk Bars, Frosted Flake	3	2.5	+
Kellogg's Cereal & Milk Bars, Froot Loops	3	2	-
Kellogg's Nutri-Grain Cereal Bars	3	0.5	+
Kellogg's Nutri-Grain Yogurt Bars, all flavors	3	0.5	+
Kellogg's Nutri-Grain Twists	3	0.5	+
Kellogg's Pop-Tarts, S'Mores	6	1	+
Kellogg's Pop-Tarts, Chocolate Chip	6	2	+
Kellogg's Pop-Tarts, Blueberry & Yogurt	6	1.5	+

CEREALS & CEREAL FOODS *(cont.)*

Food Item	Total Fat	Sat. Fat	Trans Fat
Kellogg's Pop-Tarts Pastry Swirls, Cheese Danish, Strawberry, Apple Cinnamon	11	3	+
Quaker Breakfast Squares, Baked Apple	4	1	-
Quaker Breakfast Squares, Brown Sugar Cinnamon	4	1	-
Quaker Breakfast Squares, Oatmeal Raisin	4	1	-
Quaker Chewy Dipps, Caramel Nut	6	3	+
Quaker Chewy Dipps, Chocolate Chip	6	3.5	+
Quaker Chewy Dipps, Peanut Butter	8	3	+
Quaker Chewy Granola Bar, Chocolate Chip	4	1.5	+
Quaker Chewy Granola Bars, Peanut Butter & Chocolate Chunk	3.5	1	+
Quaker Chewy Granola Bars, S'mores, Low Fat	2	0.5	+
Quaker Chewy Trail Mix Granola Bars, Chocolate, Raisin & Peanut	5	1.5	-
Quaker Chewy Trail Mix Granola Bars, Cranberry Raisin	4.5	1	-
Quaker Chewy Trail Mix Granola Bars, Mixed Nuts	6	1	-
Quaker Chewy Trail Mix Granola Bars, Tropical Fruit & Nut	4.5	1.5	-
Quaker Chewy Wholesome Favorites, Baked Apple	2	0.5	+

CEREALS & CEREAL FOODS *(cont.)*

Food Item	Total Fat	Sat. Fat	Trans Fat
Quaker Chewy Wholesome			
Favorites, Cinnamon Sugar	2	0.5	+
Quaker Fruit & Oatmeal Cereal Bars			
Iced Raspberry, Low Fat	2.5	0	-
Quaker Fruit & Oatmeal Cereal Bars			
Strawberry Cheesecake, Low Fat	3	0	-

BEST BETS: Health Valley cereal bars, granola bars, and tarts

COOKIES & CRACKERS

Food Item	Total Fat	Sat. Fat	Trans Fat
Cookies, Chocolate/Chocolate Chip			
Archway Dutch Cocoa	3.5	1	+
Archway Chocolate Chip, Sugar Free	5	1.5	+
Estee Fructose Sweetened Chocolate			
Chip	8	2	-
Estee Fructose Sweetened Chocolate			
Fudge	7	1.5	+
Keebler Chips Deluxe, Original	4.5	1.5	+
Keebler Chips Deluxe, Soft N Chewy	3	1	+
Keebler Chips Deluxe, Tropical			
Coconut	4.5	1	+
Keebler E.L. Fudge, Butterfinger			
Blasted	9	3.5	+
Keebler E.L. Fudge, Double Stuffed	9	2	+
Keebler E.L. Fudge, S'Mores Blasted	9	3.5	+

THE TRANS FAT REMEDY

COOKIES & CRACKERS *(cont.)*

Food Item	Total Fat	Sat. Fat	Trans Fat
Keebler Fudge Shoppe, Clusters Mint Creme	11	8	+
Keebler Fudge Shoppe, Clusters Peanut 'N Caramel	6	2.5	+
Keebler Fudge Shoppe, Fudge Sticks	8	4	+
Keebler Fudge Shoppe, Fudge Stripes	8	4.5	+
Keebler Fudge Shoppe, Grasshopper	7	4	+
Mother's Chocolate Chip	8	3	+
Mother's Chocolate Chip, Sugar Free	7	2	+
Mother's Chocolate Creme, Sugar Free	7	2	+
Mother's Double Fudge	9	4.5	+
Mother's Hawaiian Chocolate Chip	11	5	+
Mrs. Fields Chocolate Chip	7	4	-
Mrs. Fields Milk Chocolate Chip	8	4.5	-
Nabisco Chips Ahoy!, Candy Blasts	4	1	+
Nabisco Chips Ahoy!, Chocolate Chewy	7	2.5	+
Nabisco Chips Ahoy!, Chunky	4	1.5	-
Nabisco Chips Ahoy!, Cremewiches	7	2.5	+
Nabisco Chips Ahoy!, reduced fat	5	1.5	-
Nabisco Chips Ahoy!, Rich Chocolate	8	2.5	-
Nabisco Oreo, Chocolate Crème	7	1.5	+
Nabisco Oreo, Double Stuf	7	1.5	+
Nabisco Oreo, Fudge Covered	5	1	+

COOKIES & CRACKERS *(cont.)*

Food Item	Total Fat	Sat. Fat	Trans Fat
Nabisco Oreo, Fudge Mint Covered	4.5	1	+
Nabisco Oreo, Mint & Creme	7	1.5	+
Nabisco Oreo, Original	7	1.5	+
Nabisco Oreo, Reduced Fat	3.5	1	+
Nabisco Oreo, Uh-Oh!	7	1.5	+
SnackWell's, Chocolate Chip	4	1.5	-
SnackWell's Chocolate Chip, Sugar Free	8	2.5	+
SnackWell's Devil's Food, Fat Free	0	0	0
Sorbee, Sugar-Free Chocolate Chip	6	2.5	+
Sorbee, Sugar-Free Chocolate Fudge	6	1.5	+

BEST BET: SnackWell's Devil's Food, Fat Free. Try the Brownie recipe in chapter 6.

Cookies, Fruit

Food Item	Total Fat	Sat. Fat	Trans Fat
Archway Frosty Lemon	4	1.5	+
Archway Cherry	3	1	+
Archway Coconut Macaroon	5	4.5	0
Mother's Big Fig	1.5	0	-
Mother's Iced Lemonade	8	1.5	+
Mother's Macaroons	8	4	+
Nabisco Apple Newtons	0	0	0
Nabisco Fig Newtons, Original	2.5	0	-
Nabisco Raspberry Newtons	0	0	0
Nabisco Strawberry Newtons	1.5	0	-

BEST BETS: Nabisco Newtons, Fig, Apple and Raspberry

COOKIES & CRACKERS *(cont.)*

Food Item	Total Fat	Sat. Fat	Trans Fat
Cookies, Graham			
Keebler Fudge Shoppe, Deluxe Grahams	7	4.5	+
Keebler Grahams, Cinnamon Crisp	3	0.5	-
Keebler Grahams, Honey	4	1	-
Keebler Rumbly Grahams, Chocolate Chip	4.5	1	+
Keebler Rumbly Grahams, Cinnamon	5	1	+
Nabisco Honey Maid Graham Crackers	3	0.5	+
Nabisco Honey Maid Graham Crackers, Chocolate	3	0.5	+
Nabisco Honey Maid Graham Crackers, Low Fat	1.5	0	-
Nabisco Teddy Grahams, Chocolate	4.5	1	+
Nabisco Teddy Grahams, Chocolaty Chip	4.5	1	+
Nabisco Teddy Grahams, Cinnamon	4	1	+
Nabisco Teddy Grahams, Honey	4	1	+

BEST BETS: None. See recipes for Brownies and No-Bake Crispy Bars in chapter 6.

Food Item	Total Fat	Sat. Fat	Trans Fat
Cookies, Oatmeal			
Archway Apple Oatmeal	3	0.5	+
Archway Date Oatmeal	3	0.5	+
Archway Oatmeal Raisin	3.5	1	-

COOKIES & CRACKERS *(cont.)*

Food Item	Total Fat	Sat. Fat	Trans Fat
Estee Fructose Sweetened Oatmeal Raisin	7	1.5	+
Mother's Iced Oatmeal	4	1.5	+
Mother's Oatmeal, Sugar Free	6	1.5	+
Mother's Oatmeal Raisin	6	2	+
Mrs. Fields Oatmeal Raisin	7	3	-
SnackWell's Oatmeal, Sugar Free	2.5	0.5	+
Sorbee, Sugar-Free Oatmeal	4	1	+

BEST BETS: None. See recipes for Brownies and No-Bake Crispy Bars in chapter 6.

Cookies, Other

Food Item	Total Fat	Sat. Fat	Trans Fat
Archway Rocky Road, Sugar Free	5	1	+
Estee Fructose Sweetened Sandwich	6	1.5	+
Mother's Butter	8	3	+
Mother's English Tea	7	4	+
Mother's Taffy	8	2	+
Mother's Vanilla Cremes	7	4	+
Mrs. Fields Macadamia	8	4.5	+
Nabisco Ginger Snaps	2.5	0.5	-
SnackWell's Creme Sandwich, Sugar Free	6	1.5	+
SnackWell's, Mint Creme	3.5	1	+
Sorbee, Sugar-Free Animal	3	0.5	+

BEST BETS: None. See recipes for Brownies and No-Bake Crispy Bars in chapter 6.

COOKIES & CRACKERS *(cont.)*

Food Item	Total Fat	Sat. Fat	Trans Fat
Cookies, Peanut Butter			
Archway Peanut Butter, Sugar Free	6	1.5	+
Estee Fructose Sweetened Peanut Butter	8	1.5	-
Mother's Peanut Butter Gauchos	10	2.5	+
Nabisco Chips Ahoy!, Peanut Butter	4	1.5	+
Nabisco Nutter Butter	6	1	+
Nabisco Nutter Butter Creme Patties	10	1.5	+

BEST BETS: None. See recipes for Brownies and No-Bake Crispy Bars in chapter 6.

Cookies, Shortbread			
Estee Fructose Sweetened Shortbread	5	1	+
Keebler Sandies, Cinnamon Shortbread	5	1	+
Keebler Sandies, Pecan Shortbread	5	1	+
Keebler Sandies, Pecan Shortbread, Reduced Fat	3.5	1	+
Keebler Sandies, Simply Shortbread	4.5	2	+
Mother's Pecan Shortbread	11	2	+
Mother's Striped Shortbread	8	5	+

BEST BETS: None. See recipes for Brownies and No-Bake Crispy Bars in chapter 6.

Cookies, Wafer			
Estee Sugar-Free Creme Wafers, Strawberry or Vanilla	9	2	+

COOKIES & CRACKERS *(cont.)*

Food Item	Total Fat	Sat. Fat	Trans Fat
Keebler Vanilla Wafers	7	2	+
Mother's Checkerboard Wafers	8	2	+
Mother's Checkerboard Wafers, Sugar Free	9	2	+
Nabisco Nilla Wafers	6	1	+
Nabisco Nilla Wafers, Reduced Fat	2	0	+
Nabisco Sugar Wafers	8	1.5	+

BEST BETS: None. See recipes for Brownies and No-Bake Crispy Bars in chapter 6.

Crackers

Carr's Table Water Crackers	1.5	0	-
Dare Breton, Original	3	1.5	-
Dare Breton, Sesame Wheat	3	1.5	-
Dare Vivant, Zesty Vegetable	2.5	1.5	+
Keebler Cheese & Peanut Butter Sandwich Crackers	10	2	+
Keebler Club & Cheddar Sandwich Crackers	12	2.5	+
Keebler Club Crackers, Original	3	1	+
Keebler Club Crackers, Reduced Fat	2	0	+
Keebler Munch'ems, Cheddar	6	1.5	+
Keebler Munch'ems, Ranch	5	1	+
Keebler Scooby-Doo Baked Cheddar Crackers	7	1	+
Keebler Toast & Peanut Butter Sandwich Crackers	10	2	+

COOKIES & CRACKERS *(cont.)*

Food Item	Total Fat	Sat. Fat	Trans Fat
Keebler Toasteds, Wheat	3.5	0.5	+
Keebler Toasteds, Sesame	4	0.5	+
Keebler Townhouse, Wheat	4.5	0.5	+
Keebler Wheatables, Original	6	1	+
Nabisco, Bacon	8	1.5	+
Nabisco Better Cheddar	7	1.5	+
Nabisco Cheese Nips Crackers w/Peanut Butter, sandwich style	8	1.5	+
Nabisco Chicken in a Biskit	10	2	+
Nabisco Ritz, Garlic & Butter	4	1	+
Nabisco Ritz, Original	4	1	+
Nabisco Ritz w/Real Cheese Sandwich Crackers	12	2.5	+
Nabisco Sociables	3.5	0.5	+
Nabisco, Swiss Cheese	7	1.5	+
Nabisco Triscuits, Cheddar	5	1	+
Nabisco Triscuits, Deli Style Rye	5	1	+
Nabisco Triscuits, Garden Herb	4.5	1	+
Nabisco Triscuits, Original	5	1	+
Nabisco Triscuits, Reduced Fat	3	0.5	+
Nabisco Triscuits, Thin Crisps, French Onion	4.5	1	+
Nabisco Triscuits, Thin Crisps, Original	5	1	+
Nabisco Vegetable Thins	9	1.5	+
Nabisco Wheat Thins	6	1	+
Nabisco Wheat Thins, Harvest Crisps, Garden Vegetable	3.5	0.5	+

COOKIES & CRACKERS *(cont.)*

Food Item	Total Fat	Sat. Fat	Trans Fat
Nabisco Wheat Thins, Honey	6	1	+
Nabisco Wheat Thins, Multi-Grain	4.5	1	+
Nabisco, Wheat Thins, Reduced Fat	4	1	+
Old London Melba Snacks, White	1	0	+
Old London Melba Snacks, Sesame	3	0.5	+
Old London Melba Snacks, Garlic	1	0	+
Pepperidge Farm Goldfish, Cheddar	6	1.5	+
Pepperidge Farm Goldfish, Original	6	1.5	+
Pepperidge Farm Goldfish, Parmesan	6	1.5	+
Pepperidge Farm Goldfish, Pizza	7	1.5	+
Pepperidge Farm Sesame Snack Sticks	6	1	+
Premium Saltines, Fat Free	0	0	0
Premium Saltines, Multi-grain	1.5	0	-
Premium Saltines, Original	2	0	-
Premium Soup & Oyster Crackers	1.5	0	-
Red Oval Farm Stoned Wheat Thins	1.5	0	-
Sunshine Cheez-It	8	2	+
Sunshine Cheez-It, Reduced Fat	4.5	1	-
Sunshine Cheez-It, Sour Cream & Onion	7	1	+
Sunshine Cheez-It, White Cheddar	7	1.5	+
Zesta Saltines	1.5	0.5	+

BEST BET: Premium Saltines, Fat Free. Also see our Whole Wheat Cracker recipe in chapter 6.

DAIRY—CHEESES, MILK, YOGURT

Food Item	Total Fat	Sat. Fat	Trans Fat
Cheese (Slices, Chunks, Shredded)			
Alpine Lace Swiss Deli Sliced, Reduced Fat	7	4.5	0
Athenos Blue Cheese	10	6	0
Athenos Feta, Traditional	7	4.5	0
Athenos Feta w/Basil & Tomato	8	5	0
Athenos Feta w/Herb & Garlic	7	4.5	0
Athenos Gorgonzola	9	6	0
Borden American Singles	4.5	3	0
Borden 2% Milk Singles, American	3	2	0
Borden 2% Milk Singles, Sharp	3	2	0
Borden California Colby & Monterey Jack Chunk	9	5	0
Borden California Mild Cheddar Chunk	9	5	0
Borden California Sharp Cheddar Chunk	9	5	0
Galaxy Veggie Shreds, all flavors	3	0	0
Galaxy Veggie Slices, all flavors	3	0	0
Kraft Classic Melts, Four Cheese, Shredded	8	5	0
Kraft Cracker Barrel Cheese, Baby Swiss	9	6	0
Kraft Cracker Barrel Cheese, New York Aged Reserve	10	7	0
Kraft Cracker Barrel Cheese, Vermont Sharp White	9	6	0
Kraft Cracker Barrel Cheese, Extra Sharp	6	4	0

DAIRY—CHEESES, MILK, YOGURT *(cont.)*

Food Item	Total Fat	Sat. Fat	Trans Fat
Kraft Deli Deluxe, American Slices	7	4	0
Kraft Deli Deluxe, Sharp Cheddar Slices	9	5	0
Kraft Fat-Free, Sharp Cheddar Slices	0	0	0
Kraft Mexican Style, Four Cheese, Shredded	9	5	0
Kraft Mexican Style, Cheddar Jack, Shredded	9	5	0
Kraft Mild Mexican Slices, Singles	5	3	0
Kraft Sharp Cheddar Slices, Singles	4.5	3	0
Kraft 2% Milk Mozzarella Slices	3	2	0
Kraft 2% Milk Pepper Jack Slices	2.5	1.5	0
Kraft 2% Milk Swiss Slices	3	2	0
Kraft Velveeta Slices	4.5	2.5	0
Kraft Velveeta Slices, Extra Thick	7	4.5	0
Sargento Deli Style, Colby Slices	7	4	0
Sargento Deli Style, Medium Cheddar Slices	7	4	0
Sargento Deli Style, Mozzarella Slices	4	2.5	0
Sargento Deli Style, Muenster Slices	6	4	0
Sargento Deli Style, Provolone Slices	5	3.5	0
Sargento Deli Style, Swiss Slices	5	3	0

BEST BETS: Galaxy Veggie Shreds and Slices; Kraft Fat-Free Sharp Cheddar Slices; all Kraft 2% Milk varieties

DAIRY—CHEESES, MILK, YOGURT *(cont.)*

Food Item	Total Fat	Sat. Fat	Trans Fat
Cheese (Cottage, Ricotta)			
Frigo Ricotta, Low Fat	3	2	0
Knudsen Cottage Cheese, Traditional	5	3.5	0
Knudsen Cottage Cheese, Low Fat	2.5	1.5	0
Knudsen Cottage Cheese, Nonfat	0	0	0
Precious Low-Fat Ricotta	3	1.5	0
Precious Part Skim Ricotta	6	4	0
Precious Whole Milk Ricotta	8	5	0
Shamrock Cottage Cheese, Traditional	4.5	2.5	0
Shamrock Cottage Cheese, Low Fat	2	1.5	0
Shamrock Cottage Cheese, Nonfat	0	0	0

BEST BETS: Frigo Ricotta, Low Fat; Knudsen Cottage Cheese, Low Fat and Nonfat; Precious Ricotta, Low Fat; Shamrock Cottage Cheese, Low Fat and Nonfat

Food Item	Total Fat	Sat. Fat	Trans Fat
Cheese Spreads			
Alouette Cucumber Dill	4	2.5	0
Alouette Sun-dried Tomato & Basil	7	4.5	0
Alouette Triple Onion	7	4.5	0
Heluva Good	7	3	0
Kaukauna Lite	3.5	2	0
Kaukauna Garden Vegetable	8	5	0
Kraft Old English	8	5	0
Kraft Pineapple or Pimento	6	4	0
Kraft Roka Blue	7	5	0
Philadelphia Cream Cheese, Chive & Onion	9	6	0

DAIRY—CHEESES, MILK, YOGURT *(cont.)*

Food Item	Total Fat	Sat. Fat	Trans Fat
Philadelphia Cream Cheese, Fat Free	0	0	0
Philadelphia Cream Cheese, Garden Vegetable	9	6	0
Philadelphia Cream Cheese, Honey Nut	8	5	0
Philadelphia Cream Cheese, Light	4.5	3	0
Philadelphia Cream Cheese, Mixed Berry, whipped	6	3.5	0
Philadelphia Cream Cheese, Pineapple	8	5	0
Philadelphia Cream Cheese, Regular	9	6	0
Philadelphia Cream Cheese, Salmon	8	5	0
Rondele Bread Essentials	9	5	0
Rondele Deluxe or Regular	9	6	0
Rondele Lite	5	3	0

BEST BET: Philadelphia Cream Cheese, Fat Free.

Creamers

International Delight, all flavors	1.5	0	+
International Delight, Fat Free	0	0	0
Nestlé Coffee-Mate, all flavors	2	0	+
Nestlé Coffee-Mate, fat free	0	0	0

BEST BETS: International Delight, Fat Free; Nestlé Coffee-Mate, Fat Free

Milk

Cow's milk, 1%, all brands	2.5	1.5	0
Cow's milk, 2%, all brands	5	3	0

DAIRY—CHEESES, MILK, YOGURT *(cont.)*

Food Item	Total Fat	Sat. Fat	Trans Fat
Cow's milk, skim, all brands	0	0	0
Cow's milk, whole, all brands	8	5	0
Lactaid, Fat Free	0	0	0
Lactaid, Reduced Fat	5	3	0
Lactaid, whole milk	9	5	0
Shamrock buttermilk, 1%	2.5	1.5	0
Silk Soymilk, Chocolate	3.5	0	0
Silk Soymilk, Original	4	0	0
Silk Soymilk, Vanilla	3.5	0	0

BEST BETS: Cow's milk, 1%; Lactaid, Fat Free; Shamrock buttermilk, 1%; Silk Soymilk, all flavors

Yogurt

Food Item	Total Fat	Sat. Fat	Trans Fat
Dannon, Coffee	2.5	1.5	0
Dannon Fruit Blend, Peach	1.5	1	0
Dannon Fruit Blend, Raspberry	2	1	0
Dannon, La Creme Mousse, Strawberry	5	3.5	0
Dannon Light 'N Fit, all flavors	0	0	0
Mountain Dairy, Low Fat, all flavors	1.5	1	0
Yoplait Light, Fat Free, all flavors	0	0	0
Yoplait Nouriche, all flavors	0	0	0
Yoplait Original, 99% Fat Free, all flavors	1.5	1	0
Yoplait Whips, all flavors	2.5	2	0

BEST BETS: Dannon Light 'N Fit, all flavors; Yoplait Light, Fat Free, all flavors; Yoplait Nouriche, all flavors

DINNER MIXES—DRY, BOXED

Note: This category consists of items that typically contain an entire entrée (or, in some cases, an entire meal) in a box, or require the addition of meat or poultry, with minimal preparation. Some products are pasta-based; others focus on meat or poultry.

Food Item	Total Fat	Sat. Fat	Trans Fat
Banquet Homestyle Bakes, Beef, Chili & Beans, prepared	11	4	-
Banquet Homestyle Bakes, Creamy Chicken & Biscuits, prepared	16	3.5	-
Banquet Homestyle Bakes, Creamy Turkey & Stuffing, prepared	15	3.5	0
Banquet Homestyle Bakes, Dumplings & Chicken, prepared	9	2.5	-
Banquet Homestyle Bakes, Italian Pasta w/Meatballs & Garlic Bread, prepared	16	5	-
Banquet Homestyle Bakes, Pizza Pasta, prepared	7	1.5	-
Betty Crocker Complete Meals, Ham & Au Gratin Potatoes	13	4.5	-
Betty Crocker Complete Meals, Homestyle Dumplings & Chicken	9	3	-
Betty Crocker Complete Meals, Lasagna w/Meat Sauce	8	3	-
Betty Crocker Hamburger Helper, Beef & Garlic Potatoes, prepared	13	5	-

DINNER MIXES—DRY, BOXED *(cont.)*

Food Item	Total Fat	Sat. Fat	Trans Fat
Betty Crocker Hamburger Helper, Beef Pasta, prepared	13	5	-
Betty Crocker Hamburger Helper, Cheeseburger Macaroni, prepared	16	6	+
Betty Crocker Hamburger Helper, Cheesy Baked Potato, prepared	15	6	+
Betty Crocker Hamburger Helper, Cheesy Enchilada, prepared	15	6	+
Betty Crocker Hamburger Helper, Cheesy Hashbrowns, prepared	20	7	+
Betty Crocker Hamburger Helper, Lasagna, prepared	12	4.5	-
Betty Crocker Hamburger Helper, Potatoes Stroganoff, prepared	13	5	+
Betty Crocker Hamburger Helper, Ravioli & Cheese, prepared	12	5	-
Betty Crocker Pork Helper, Pork Chops & Stuffing, prepared	14	4	-
Betty Crocker Pork Helper, Pork Fried Rice, prepared	15	4	0
Betty Crocker Tuna Helper, Au Gratin, prepared	12	3	+
Betty Crocker Tuna Helper, Cheesy Pasta, prepared	11	3	+

DINNER MIXES—DRY, BOXED *(cont.)*

Food Item	Total Fat	Sat. Fat	Trans Fat
Betty Crocker Tuna Helper, Creamy Broccoli, prepared	13	3.5	+
Betty Crocker Tuna Helper, Creamy Pasta, prepared	13	3.5	+
Betty Crocker Tuna Helper, Fettuccine Alfredo, prepared	14	4	+
Campbell's Supper Bakes, Cheesy Chicken, prepared	10	5	-
Campbell's Supper Bakes, Herb Chicken, prepared	7	3.5	-
Campbell's Supper Bakes, Lemon Chicken, prepared	7	3.5	-
Campbell's Supper Bakes, Savory Pork Chops, prepared	18	7	-

BEST BETS: None. Try some of the delicious recipes in chapter 6.

DIPS, DRESSINGS & OILS

Food Item	Total Fat	Sat. Fat	Trans Fat
Dips/Spreads			
Athenos Hummus, Artichoke & Garlic	2.5	0	0
Athenos Hummus, Cucumber Dill	3	0	0
Athenos Hummus, Original	3	0	0

DIPS, DRESSINGS & OILS *(cont.)*

Food Item	Total Fat	Sat. Fat	Trans Fat
Athenos Hummus, Roasted Garlic	3	0	0
Dean's French Onion Dip, refrigerated	4.5	0.5	+
Dean's Ranch Dip, refrigerated	5	1	+
Dean's Zesty Guacamole Dip, refrigerated	9	3	+
Kraft Cheez Whiz, Light	3.5	2	0
Kraft Cheez Whiz, Original	7	2.5	+
Kraft Cheez Whiz, Salsa con Queso	3	1	+
Kraft Easy Cheese, American, aerosol can	6	4	0
Kraft Easy Cheese, Nacho, aerosol can	7	4.5	0
Kraft Easy Cheese, Sharp Cheddar, aerosol can	6	4	0
Kraft Velveeta, Light	3	2	0
Kraft Velveeta, Original	6	4	0
Lakeview Farms Bacon & Onion Dip, refrigerated	3.5	0.5	+
Lakeview Farms Guacamole Dip, refrigerated	3.5	0.5	+
Lakeview Farms Ranch Dip, refrigerated	3.5	0.5	+
Pace Salsa con Queso	3	1	+
Price's French Onion Dip, refrigerated	5	3	0
Price's Green Chili Dip, refrigerated	5	3	0

DIPS, DRESSINGS & OILS *(cont.)*

Food Item	Total Fat	Sat. Fat	Trans Fat
Price's Jalapeno Dip, refrigerated	5	3	0
Price's Red Chili Dip, refrigerated	5	3	0

BEST BETS: Athenos Hummus, all; Kraft Cheez Whiz, Light; Kraft Velveeta, Light

Dressings (Nonrefrigerated)

Food Item	Total Fat	Sat. Fat	Trans Fat
Annie's Naturals Balsamic Vinaigrette	10	0.5	0
Annie's Naturals Cowgirl Ranch	11	1	0
Annie's Naturals Goddess Dressing	13	1	0
Annie's Naturals Organic Thousand Island	7	1	0
Annie's Naturals Roasted Red Pepper Vinaigrette	6	0.5	0
Annie's Naturals Shiitake & Sesame Vinaigrette	13	1	0
Bernstein's Balsamic Italian	11	0.5	0
Bernstein's Cheese Fantastico Light	1.5	0.5	0
Bernstein's Cheese & Garlic Italian	11	1	0
Bernstein's Cheese & Garlic Italian, Fat Free	0	0	0
Bernstein's Red Wine & Garlic	11	1	0
Bernstein's Restaurant Recipe Italian	12	1	0
Best Foods Just2Good Mayonnaise	2	0.5	0
Best Foods Real Mayonnaise	11	1.5	0
Emeril's Bacon Vinaigrette	10	1	0
Emeril's Caesar	14	1	0

DIPS, DRESSINGS & OILS *(cont.)*

Food Item	Total Fat	Sat. Fat	Trans Fat
Emeril's Honey Mustard	9	0.5	0
Emeril's House Herb Vinaigrette	10	0.5	0
Emeril's Romano	12	1	0
Girard's Blue Cheese Vinaigrette	10	2	0
Girard's Caesar	15	2.5	0
Girard's Champagne	16	2.5	0
Girard's Honey Dijon Peppercorn	13	2	0
Girard's Old Venice Italian	13	2	0
Girard's Raspberry	10	1.5	0
Girard's Spinach Salad	2	0	0
Hidden Valley BBQ Ranch	12	2	0
Hidden Valley Ranch	14	2.5	0
Hidden Valley Ranch w/Bacon	14	2.5	0
Hidden Valley Ranch, Light	7	1	0
Hollywood Safflower Mayonnaise	11	1.5	0
Kraft Caesar, Fat Free	0	0	0
Kraft Caesar, Italian w/Oregano	10	1.5	-
Kraft Catalina	6	1	0
Kraft Light Done Right, Italian	3	0.5	0
Kraft Light Done Right, Ranch	4.5	0.5	0
Kraft Light Done Right, Raspberry Vinaigrette	4	0	0
Kraft Mayonnaise	11	1.5	0
Kraft Miracle Whip, Light	2	0	0
Kraft Miracle Whip, Nonfat	0	0	0
Kraft Miracle Whip, Original	4	0.5	0
Kraft Ranch, Fat Free	0	0	0

DIPS, DRESSINGS & OILS *(cont.)*

Food Item	Total Fat	Sat. Fat	Trans Fat
Kraft Seven Seas, Red Wine Vinaigrette	9	0.5	0
Kraft Seven Seas, Viva Italian	9	1	0
Kraft Thousand Island	6	1	0
Kraft Three Cheese Ranch	18	3	0
Kraft Zesty Italian	8	1	0
Newman's Own Balsamic Vinaigrette	9	1	0
Newman's Own Creamy Caesar	18	3	0
Newman's Own Family Recipe Italian	13	1	0
Newman's Own Light Raspberry & Walnut	5	0.5	0
Newman's Own Parmesan & Roasted Garlic	11	2	0
Newman's Own Ranch	15	2	0
Wish-Bone Blue Cheese, Chunky	17	3	+
Wish-Bone Creamy Caesar	18	3	0
Wish-Bone 5 Cheese Italian	10	1.5	0
Wish-Bone Deluxe, French	11	1.5	0
Wish-Bone French, Sweet 'n Spicy	12	2	0
Wish-Bone House Berry Vinaigrette	4.5	0.5	0
Wish-Bone Italian Dressing	8	1	0
Wish-Bone Just2Good, Honey Dijon	2	0	0
Wish-Bone Just2Good, Italian	2	0	0
Wish-Bone Just2Good, Ranch	2	0	0
Wish-Bone Ranch Dressing	17	2.5	0
Wish-Bone Ranch Up! Cheese	16	2.5	0

DIPS, DRESSINGS & OILS *(cont.)*

Food Item	Total Fat	Sat. Fat	Trans Fat
Wish-Bone Ranch Up! Classic	15	2	0
Wish-Bone Ranch Up! Zesty	15	2	0
Wish-Bone Spring Onion Ranch	14	2	0
Wish-Bone Thousand Island	12	2	0

BEST BETS: Bernstein's Cheese & Garlic Italian, Fat Free; Bernstein's Cheese Fantastico, Light; Best Foods Just2Good Mayonnaise; Girard Spinach Salad; Kraft Caesar, Fat Free; Kraft Miracle Whip, Nonfat; Kraft Ranch, Fat Free; Wish-Bone Just2Good, all. Also try the Lite Thousand Island Dressing in chapter 6.

Dressings (Refrigerated)

Lighthouse Bleu Cheese	16	1.5	0
Lighthouse Caesar	14	1.5	0
Lighthouse Cole Slaw	7	0.5	0
Lighthouse Poppyseed	12	1	0
Lighthouse Ranch	12	1	0
Marie's Blue Cheese	19	3.5	0
Marie's Caesar	19	3	0
Marie's Cole Slaw	13	2	0
Marie's Creamy Ranch	19	3	0
Marie's Jalapeno Ranch	17	2.5	0
Marie's Poppy Seed	13	2	0

BEST BETS: None. Select one of the Best Bets from the nonrefrigerated dressings list instead.

Oils

Bertolli Extra Light Olive Oil	14	2	0
Bertolli Extra Virgin Olive Oil	14	2	0

DIPS, DRESSINGS & OILS *(cont.)*

Food Item	Total Fat	Sat. Fat	Trans Fat
Canola Harvest	14	1	0
GrapeOla Oil	14	1	0
Hollywood Safflower Oil	14	1	0
Hollywood Peanut Oil	14	2	0
Mazola Corn Oil	14	2	0
Mazola Canola Oil	14	1	0
Mazola Vegetable Oil	14	2	0
Wesson Canola	14	1	0
Wesson Best Blend	14	1.5	0
Wesson Vegetable Oil	14	2	0

BEST BET: Bertolli olive oils, because of the high monounsaturated (healthy fat) level

FROZEN FOODS—BREAKFAST

Food Item	Total Fat	Sat. Fat	Trans Fat
Entrées			
Amy's Breakfast Burrito, Organic	6	<1	0
Jimmy Dean Biscuit Sandwich, Bacon, Egg & Cheese	15	5	+
Jimmy Dean Biscuit Sandwich, Sausage	28	9	+
Jimmy Dean Biscuit Sandwich, Sausage, Egg & Cheese	24	8	+
Lightlife Smart Links (nonmeat sausages)	2	0	0
Pillsbury Toaster Scrambles, Cheese, Egg & Bacon	12	3.5	+

FROZEN FOODS—BREAKFAST *(cont.)*

Food Item	Total Fat	Sat. Fat	Trans Fat
Pillsbury Toaster Scrambles, Cheese, Egg & Sausage	12	3.5	+
Red Baron Western Scramble Breakfast Singles	19	6	-
Swanson Great Starts, Breakfast Wrap w/Bacon	11	4	+
Swanson Great Starts, Eggs & Bacon	22	8	-
Swanson Great Starts, Egg, Ham & Cheese on Bagel	12	4.5	0
Swanson Great Starts, Eggs & Sausage	27	9	-
Swanson Great Starts, French Toast & Sausage	25	10	-
Swanson Great Starts, Pancakes & Sausage	25	11	-
Swanson Great Starts, Sausage, Egg & Cheese on Croissant	33	11	+
Swanson Hungry Man All-Day Breakfast	64	21	-
Uncle Ben's Breakfast Bowl, Apple & Cinnamon Pancakes	8	4.5	0
Uncle Ben's Breakfast Bowl, Bacon, Egg & Potatoes	13	6	0
Uncle Ben's Breakfast Bowl, Egg, Cheese & Salsa	21	4	0
Uncle Ben's Breakfast Bowl, French Toast & Sausage	22	7	+

FROZEN FOODS—BREAKFAST *(cont.)*

Food Item	Total Fat	Sat. Fat	Trans Fat
Uncle Ben's Breakfast Bowl, Ham, Egg & Peppers	9	4.5	0
Uncle Ben's Breakfast Bowl, Sausage, Egg & Biscuit	20	8	0

BEST BET: Lightlife Smart Links. Enjoy them with the Apple Waffle recipe in chapter 6 or Ore-Ida Hash Browns (see "Frozen Foods," Potatoes/Onion Rings).

French Toast, Waffles, Pancakes, Strudel

Food Item	Total Fat	Sat. Fat	Trans Fat
Aunt Jemima Buttermilk Waffles	3	0.5	+
Farm Rich French Toast Sticks, Cinnamon	15	2.5	-
Farm Rich French Toast Sticks, Original	12	2	-
Kashi GoLean Blueberry Waffles	3	0	0
Kashi GoLean Original Waffles	3	0	0
Kellogg's Eggo Buttermilk Waffles	7	1.5	+
Kellogg's Eggo Apple Cinnamon Waffles	7	1.5	+
Kellogg's Eggo Cinnamon Toast Waffles	10	2.5	+
Kellogg's Eggo Chocolate Chip Waffles	7	1.5	+
Kellogg's Eggo Homestyle Waffles	7	1.5	+
Krusteaz Buttermilk Pancakes	4	1	0
Krusteaz Cinnamon Swirl French Toast	5	1	-

FROZEN FOODS—BREAKFAST *(cont.)*

Food Item	Total Fat	Sat. Fat	Trans Fat
Pillsbury Pancakes, Buttermilk	4	1	-
Pillsbury Toaster Strudel, Apple	8	1.5	+
Pillsbury Toaster Strudel, Cherry	8	1.5	+
Pillsbury Toaster Strudel, Strawberry	8	2	+
Pillsbury Waffle Sticks, Blueberry	7	2	+
Pillsbury Waffle Sticks, Homestyle	6	2	+

BEST BET: Kashi GoLean Waffles; also try the Apple Waffle recipe in chapter 6.

FROZEN FOODS—DAIRY

Food Item	Total Fat	Sat. Fat	Trans Fat
Bars/Cups/Sandwiches			
Blue Bunny Black Raspberry Ice Cream Bar	16	11	-
Blue Bunny Champs! Vanilla Ice Cream Cones	18	11	-
Blue Bunny Heath Ice Cream Bar	13	10	+
Blue Bunny Sundae Cups	5	3.5	-
Blue Bunny Sweet Freedom Vanilla Sundae Cones, No Sugar Added	13	9	-
Blue Bunny Vanilla Ice Cream Sandwich	7	3.5	-
Carvel Flying Saucer Ice Cream Sandwich	10	5	-

FROZEN FOODS—DAIRY *(cont.)*

Food Item	Total Fat	Sat. Fat	Trans Fat
Carvel Flying Saucer Ice Cream Sandwich, 98% Fat Free	1.5	0	-
Dove Milk Chocolate w/Almonds	18	10	0
Dove Milk Chocolate w/Vanilla Ice Cream	17	11	0
Dove Original Chocolate w/Chocolate Ice Cream	17	10	0
Good Humor Chocolate Eclair, on stick	8	3	-
Good Humor Strawberry Shortcake, on stick	9	2.5	-
Good Humor Toasted Almond, on stick	10	2.5	-
Häagen-Dazs Chocolate & Dark Chocolate Ice Cream Bar	20	12	0
Häagen-Dazs Raspberry Cheesecake Bar	22	13	0
Häagen-Dazs Vanilla & Milk Chocolate Ice Cream Bar	20	12	0
Healthy Choice Fudge Bars	1	0.5	0
Healthy Choice Strawberry & Cream Bar	1.5	1	0
Klondike Big Bear Vanilla Ice Cream Sandwich	7	4	-
Klondike Caramel & Peanut Ice Cream Bar	19	12	0
Klondike Heath Ice Cream Bar	20	14	+
Klondike Krunch Ice Cream Bar	19	14	0

FROZEN FOODS—DAIRY *(cont.)*

Food Item	Total Fat	Sat. Fat	Trans Fat
Klondike Oreo Ice Cream Cookie Sandwich	9	3.5	+
Klondike Slim-A-Bear, 98% Fat Free Vanilla	1.5	0	-
Klondike York Ice Cream Bar	19	13	0
Nestlé Butterfinger Ice Cream Bar	15	10	+
Nestlé Drumstick Sundae, Vanilla	21	11	+
Nestlé Drumstick Sundae, Chocolate	23	12	+
Nestlé Drumstick Sundae, Cookies & Cream	19	13	+
Slim-Fast Chocolate Fudge Bar	1.5	1	0
Starbucks Frappuccino, Java Fudge Ice Cream Bar	2	1	0
Starbucks Frappuccino, Mocha Ice Cream Bar	2	1	0

BEST BETS: Carvel Flying Saucers, 98% Fat Free; Starbucks Frappuccino, Java Fudge and Mocha; Healthy Choice Fudge Bars and Strawberry & Cream Bars; Slim-Fast Chocolate Fudge Bar

Ice Cream

Ben & Jerry's, Cherry Garcia	16	11	0
Ben & Jerry's, Cherry Garcia, Low Fat	3	2	0
Ben & Jerry's, Chocolate	16	11	0
Ben & Jerry's, Chocolate Chip Cookie Dough	15	10	-
Ben & Jerry's, Chocolate Fudge Brownie, Low Fat	2.5	1	-

FROZEN FOODS—DAIRY *(cont.)*

Food Item	Total Fat	Sat. Fat	Trans Fat
Ben & Jerry's, Chunky Monkey	19	11	0
Ben & Jerry's, New York Super Fudge Chunk	20	11	0
Ben & Jerry's, Phish Food	13	10	0
Ben & Jerry's, Peanut Butter Cup	26	13	-
Ben & Jerry's, Pistachio Pistachio	11	10	0
Ben & Jerry's, Vanilla	16	11	0
Ben & Jerry's, Vanilla Heath Bar Crunch	19	11	+
Blue Bunny, Cookies & Cream	8	4.5	-
Blue Bunny, Double Strawberry	7	4.5	0
Blue Bunny, Exquisite Mint	9	6	-
Blue Bunny, Homemade Chocolate	8	5	0
Blue Bunny, Homemade Vanilla	8	5	0
Blue Bunny, New York Cherry Cheesecake	8	4.5	-
Blue Bunny, Peanut Butter Panic	13	6	-
Blue Bunny, Praline Pecan	9	5	0
Breyers, Butter Pecan	11	5	0
Breyers, Cherry Vanilla	8	5	0
Breyers, Cookies & Cream	9	6	0
Breyers, Natural Vanilla	9	5	0
Breyers, Peach	6	4	0
Breyers, Rocky Road	8	5	0
Breyers, Vanilla & Chocolate Fudge Checks	9	5	0
Breyers, Vanilla Fudge Brownie	9	5	0
Breyers Carb Smart, Chocolate	10	6	0

FROZEN FOODS—DAIRY *(cont.)*

Food Item	Total Fat	Sat. Fat	Trans Fat
Breyers Carb Smart, Strawberry	9	6	0
Breyers Carb Smart, Vanilla	9	6	0
Breyers Ice Cream Parlor, Oreo	8	4.5	-
Breyers Ice Cream Parlor, Reese's	9	4.5	0
Dreyer's Dreamery, Banana Split	11	7	0
Dreyer's Dreamery, Brownie Turtle Sundae	17	8	-
Dreyer's Dreamery, Coney Island Waffle Cone	18	12	0
Dreyer's Dreamery, Fortunate Vanilla	17	11	0
Dreyer's Dreamery, Strawberry Fields	12	7	0
Dreyer's Dreamery, Triple Butter Pecan	18	8	0
Dreyer's Dreamery, Ultimate Mudslide	15	9	0
Dreyer's Grand, Chocolate	8	5	0
Dreyer's Grand, Cookie Dough	9	6	+
Dreyer's Grand, Cookies 'N Cream	8	4.5	-
Dreyer's Grand, French Vanilla	9	5	0
Dreyer's Grand, French Vanilla Fudge Pie	8	4.5	-
Dreyer's Grand, Mint Chocolate Chip	9	6	-
Dreyer's Grand, Real Strawberry	6	4	0
Dreyer's Grand, Rocky Road	4	2	-
Dreyer's Grand, Triple Chocolate Thunder	9	6	0
Dreyer's Grand, Ultimate Caramel Chip	8	5	-

FROZEN FOODS—DAIRY *(cont.)*

Food Item	Total Fat	Sat. Fat	Trans Fat
Dreyer's Grand, Light, Chocolate Fudge Check	4	2.5	-
Dreyer's Grand, Light, French Silk	4.5	3	-
Dreyer's Grand, Light, Strawberry Cheesecake Delight	4	2.5	-
Dreyer's Grand, Light, Vanilla	3.5	2	0
Dreyer's Grand, Light, Vanilla Raspberry Escape	3.5	2.5	-
Edy's M&M's Vanilla	9	5	+
Edy's M&M's Mint	11	6	0
Edy's Snickers Cruncher	9	5	-
Edy's Twix Peanut Butter	11	5	-
Godiva Ice Cream, Belgian Dark Chocolate	17	10	-
Godiva, Chocolate Cheesecake	17	10	-
Godiva, Chocolate w/Chocolate Hearts	20	13	0
Godiva, Chocolate Raspberry Truffle	16	9	-
Godiva, Vanilla Chocolate Raspberry	12	7	0
Godiva, Vanilla w/Chocolate Caramel Hearts	18	11	0
Häagen-Dazs, Butter Pecan	23	11	0
Häagen-Dazs, Cherry Vanilla	15	9	0
Häagen-Dazs, Chocolate	18	11	0
Häagen-Dazs, Chocolate Chocolate Chip	20	12	0
Häagen-Dazs, Cookie Dough Chip	20	12	0
Häagen-Dazs, Cookies & Cream	17	10	0

FROZEN FOODS—DAIRY *(cont.)*

Food Item	Total Fat	Sat. Fat	Trans Fat
Häagen-Dazs, Strawberry	16	10	0
Häagen-Dazs, Vanilla Fudge	18	12	0
Häagen-Dazs Desserts Extraordinaire, Bananas Foster	15	9	0
Häagen-Dazs Desserts Extraordinaire, Café Mocha Frappé	19	12	0
Häagen-Dazs Desserts Extraordinaire, Chocolate Raspberry Torte	15	9	0
Healthy Choice, Chocolate Chocolate Chunk	2	1	-
Healthy Choice, Chocolate Fudge Brownie, No Sugar Added	2	1	-
Healthy Choice, Mint Chocolate Chip	2	1	-
Healthy Choice, Mint Chocolate Chip, No Sugar Added	2	1	-
Healthy Choice, Rocky Road	2	1	-
Healthy Choice, Tin Roof Sundae	2	1	-
Healthy Choice, Vanilla	2	1	0
Healthy Choice, Vanilla, No Sugar Added	2	1	0
Shamrock Farms Homemade, Banana Split	7	4.5	0
Shamrock Farms Homemade, Milk Chocolate	9	6	0
Shamrock Farms Homemade, Old Fashioned Vanilla	9	6	0

FROZEN FOODS—DAIRY *(cont.)*

Food Item	Total Fat	Sat. Fat	Trans Fat
Shamrock Farms Homemade, Peaches & Cream	7	4.5	0

BEST BETS: Healthy Choice Vanilla and Vanilla, No Sugar Added; Ben & Jerry's Cherry Garcia, Low Fat

Sherbet/Sorbet/Yogurt (Frozen)

Food Item	Total Fat	Sat. Fat	Trans Fat
Dreyer's Key Lime Sherbet	1.5	0.5	0
Dreyer's Orange Cream Sherbet, Lite	2	1	0
Dreyer's Swiss Orange Sherbet	3	2.5	-
Dreyer's Whole Fruit Sorbet, all flavors	0	0	0
Dreyer's Heath Toffee Crunch Frozen Yogurt	4	2	-
Dreyer's Vanilla Frozen Yogurt	3.5	2.5	0
Häagen-Dazs Chocolate Fudge Brownie Frozen Yogurt, Low Fat	2.5	1.5	0
Häagen-Dazs Sorbet, Fat Free, all flavors	0	0	0
Häagen-Dazs Vanilla Frozen Yogurt	4.5	2.5	0

BEST BETS: Dreyer's Key Lime and Orange Cream sherbet; Dreyer's Whole Fruit Sorbet; Häagen-Dazs sorbet

FROZEN FOODS—DESSERTS

Food Item	Total Fat	Sat. Fat	Trans Fat
Cakes			
Edwards Pecan Cheesecake Singles	19	6	+
Essensia Delectable Cheesecake	28	15	+

FROZEN FOODS—DESSERTS *(cont.)*

Food Item	Total Fat	Sat. Fat	Trans Fat
Essensia New York Style Cheesecake	31	17	-
Mrs. Smith's Carrot Cake	16	3.5	+
Mrs. Smith's Flip It Cake, Apple Caramel	13	2	+
Mrs. Smith's Flip It Cake, Chocolate Caramel	25	7	-
Mrs. Smith's Flip It Cake, Strawberry Delight	9	1.5	+
Pepperidge Farm 3-Layer Cake, Chocolate Fudge	11	3	+
Pepperidge Farm 3-Layer Cake, Chocolate Fudge Stripe	13	3	+
Pepperidge Farm 3-Layer Cake, Coconut	11	3	+
Pepperidge Farm 3-Layer Cake, Red, White & Blue	11	2.5	+
Sara Lee All Butter Pound Cake	15	8	0
Sara Lee French Cheesecake	25	16	+
Sara Lee New York Style Cheesecake	21	11	-
Sara Lee Original Cream Cheesecake, Cherry	12	5	-
Sara Lee Original Cream Cheesecake, Classic	18	9	-
Sara Lee Original Cream Cheesecake, Strawberry	12	5	-

BEST BETS: None. Try the Chocolate Pudding and Brownie recipes in chapter 6.

FROZEN FOODS—DESSERTS *(cont.)*

Food Item	Total Fat	Sat. Fat	Trans Fat
Pies			
Edwards Key Lime Pie Singles	16	10	+
Edwards Lemon Meringue Pie	8	3	-
Edwards Lemon Meringue Singles	7	2	-
Edwards Mocha Mudslide Pie	24	12	+
Edwards Turtle Pie Singles	16	7	+
Marie Callender's Banana Cream Pie	18	8	+
Marie Callender's Cherry Crunch Cobbler	18	4.5	-
Marie Callender's Cherry Crunch Pie	15	3	-
Marie Callender's Coconut Cream Pie	20	10	+
Marie Callender's Dutch Apple Pie	16	2.5	-
Marie Callender's Lattice Apple Pie	18	2.5	-
Marie Callender's Lattice Peach Pie	20	3	-
Marie Callender's Peach Cobbler	22	3	-
Marie Callender's Raspberry Pie	20	3	-
Mrs. Smith's Blackberry Cobbler	10	2	-
Mrs. Smith's Boston Cream Pie	9	2	+
Mrs. Smith's Cream Pie	29	15	+
Sara Lee Apple Pie	16	3.5	-
Sara Lee Caramel Applenut Pie	18	4.5	+
Sara Lee Cherry Pie	14	2.5	-
Sara Lee Peach Pie	13	4	+
Sara Lee Pumpkin Pie	9	2.5	-
Sara Lee Southern Pecan Pie	24	4.5	+

BEST BETS: None. Try the Apple Pie and Blueberry Pie recipes in chapter 6.

FROZEN FOODS—DESSERTS *(cont.)*

Food Item	Total Fat	Sat. Fat	Trans Fat
Other			
Rich's Bavarian Cappuccino Eclairs	12	10	+
Rich's Bavarian Creme Eclairs	12	10	+
Sara Lee Deluxe Cinnamon Rolls	15	9	0
Sara Lee French Style Croissants	11	4	+

BEST BETS: None. Try the Brownie, Apple Pie, Blueberry Pie, and Chocolate Pudding recipes in chapter 6.

FROZEN FOODS—DINNERS, ENTRÉES, SIDES

Food Item	Total Fat	Sat. Fat	Trans Fat
Asian			
Cascadian Farm Japanese Noodles & Vegetables	2.5	0	0
Budget Gourmet Chinese Vegetables & White Chicken	7	1	-
Budget Gourmet Stir Fry Rice & Vegetables	19	3.5	+
Healthy Choice Chicken Teriyaki Dinner	6	2	-
Michelina's Yu Sing Bowls, Sesame Chicken	6	1	-
Michelina's Yu Sing Bowls, Shrimp Fried Rice	7	1	0

FROZEN FOODS—DINNERS, ENTRÉES, SIDES *(cont.)*

Food Item	Total Fat	Sat. Fat	Trans Fat
Michelina's Yu Sing Bowls, Teriyaki Chicken	3	0.5	0
Stouffer's Lean Cuisine Café Classics, Thai Style Chicken	4.5	2.5	0
Weight Watchers Smart Ones, Chicken Stir Fry Bowl	6	1.5	0
Weight Watchers Smart Ones, Teriyaki Chicken Vegetable Bowl	3	1	-
Weight Watchers Smart Ones, Thai Chicken & Rice Noodles	4	0.5	0

BEST BETS: Cascadian Farm Japanese Noodles & Vegetables; Michelina's Yu Sing Bowls, Teriyaki Chicken

Beef/Pork

Food Item	Total Fat	Sat. Fat	Trans Fat
Banquet Boneless Pork Rib Meal	20	8	+
Banquet Chicken Fried Beef Steak	23	8	+
Banquet Country Fried Pork Meal	24	7	+
Banquet Salisbury Steak Meal	20	9	-
Banquet Sliced Beef Meal	10	4.5	+
Budget Gourmet Premium, Beef Pepper Steak	4.5	1.5	0
Budget Gourmet Premium, Roast Beef Supreme	10	4	-
Budget Gourmet Premium, Swedish Meatballs	28	11	-
Healthy Choice Beef Merlot	8	2	-
Healthy Choice Beef Stroganoff	9	3	-

FROZEN FOODS—DINNERS, ENTRÉES, SIDES *(cont.)*

Food Item	Total Fat	Sat. Fat	Trans Fat
Healthy Choice Grilled Steak in Garlic Sauce	7	2.5	-
Healthy Choice Grilled Whiskey Steak	5	2	-
Healthy Choice Meat Loaf Dinner	9	3	-
Healthy Choice Salisbury Steak Dinner	9	3.5	-
Marie Callender's Beef Salisbury Steak Meal	21	11	-
Marie Callender's Meat Loaf Meal	25	12	-
Michael Angelo's Beef Cacciatore	15	2	0
Michelina's Homestyle Bowls, Vegetable & Beef Stew	6	1.5	+
Michelina's Salisbury Steak	16	7	-
OnCor Salisbury Steak & Gravy	13	6	-
Stouffer's Lean Cuisine Café Classics, Beef Portabello	7	3	0
Stouffer's Lean Cuisine Café Classics, Honey Roasted Pork	4	1.5	+
Stouffer's Lean Cuisine Café Classics, Meatloaf	8	3	0
Stouffer's Lean Cuisine Everyday Favorites, Swedish Meatballs	7	3	0
Swanson American Recipes, Beef Pot Roast	9	3	-
Swanson Hungry Man Steakhouse, Country Fried Beef Steak	29	10	+

FROZEN FOODS—DINNERS, ENTRÉES, SIDES *(cont.)*

Food Item	Total Fat	Sat. Fat	Trans Fat
Weight Watchers Smart Ones, Peppercorn Filet Beef	8	2	-
Weight Watchers Smart Ones, Roast Beef & Gravy	7	2.5	-

BEST BET: Budget Gourmet Premium, Beef Pepper Steak

Food Item	Total Fat	Sat. Fat	Trans Fat
Burgers			
Amy's American Burger	3	0	0
Amy's California Burger	5	0.5	0
Amy's Chicago Burger	5	1.5	0
Amy's Texas Burger	2.5	0	0
Boca Burger, Original Vegan	1	0	0
Gardenburger, Original	3	1.5	0
Gardenburger, Flame Grilled	4	0	0
Lightlife Light Burgers	1	0	0
Morningstar Garden Veggie Patties	2.5	0.5	0
Morningstar Grillers, Original	6	1	0
Morningstar Grilled Prime Burgers	9	1	0
Morningstar Tomato & Basil Pizza Burger	6	1.5	0
White Castle Cheeseburger	17	9	-

BEST BETS: Amy's American Burger and Texas Burger; Boca Burger, Original Vegan; Gardenburger, Original; Lightlife Light Burgers; Morningstar Garden Veggie Patties

FROZEN FOODS—DINNERS, ENTRÉES, SIDES *(cont.)*

Food Item	Total Fat	Sat. Fat	Trans Fat
Chicken/Turkey			
Banquet BBQ Chicken Meal	13	3	+
Banquet Chicken Breast Tenders	19	5	+
Banquet Chicken Fingers Meal	30	8	+
Banquet Chicken Nugget Meal	21	5	+
Banquet Chicken Patties, Original	17	3.5	+
Banquet Crispy Chicken, Country	14	3.5	+
Banquet Crispy Chicken, Southern	18	6	+
Banquet Fried Chicken Meal	27	9	+
Banquet Roasted White Turkey Meal	6	2	-
Banquet Turkey Meal	13	3.5	+
Budget Gourmet Premium, French Recipe Chicken	7	2	0
Budget Gourmet Premium, Orange Glazed Chicken	3	0.5	0
Cascadian Farm Orange Dijon Chicken	3	1	0
Healthy Choice Chicken Tuscany	9	3	-
Healthy Choice Grilled Basil Chicken	7	2.5	0
Healthy Choice Grilled Chicken Breast & Pasta	7	2.5	-
Healthy Choice Grilled Chicken Marinara	4.5	1.5	0
Healthy Choice Princess Chicken	7	2	-
Healthy Choice Traditional Turkey Breast	5	2	-

FROZEN FOODS—DINNERS, ENTRÉES, SIDES *(cont.)*

Food Item	Total Fat	Sat. Fat	Trans Fat
Healthy Choice Turkey Breast & Mashed Potatoes	7	1.5	-
Marie Callender's Baked Chicken Breast Meal	10	4.5	-
Michael Angelo's Chicken Capri	15	3	0
Michelina's Homestyle Bowls, Chicken Alfredo w/Broccoli	21	10	-
Morningstar Chik Patties, Original	6	1	0
Morningstar Parmesan Ranch Chik Patties	7	1	0
OnCor Sliced Turkey & Gravy	4	1	0
Stouffer's Chicken à La King	11	3.5	0
Stouffer's Chicken & Broccoli Pasta Bake, Family Style	15	6	-
Stouffer's Homestyle Entrées, Baked Chicken Breast	11	3	-
Stouffer's Homestyle Entrées, Chicken Parmesan	17	4	-
Stouffer's Lean Cuisine Café Classics, Chicken w/Almonds	4.5	0.5	0
Stouffer's Lean Cuisine Café Classics, Chicken Carbonara	7	2	0
Stouffer's Lean Cuisine Café Classics, Chicken in Wine Sauce	5	2	-
Stouffer's Lean Cuisine Café Classics, Glazed Chicken	5	1	0

FROZEN FOODS—DINNERS, ENTRÉES, SIDES *(cont.)*

Food Item	Total Fat	Sat. Fat	Trans Fat
Stouffer's Lean Cuisine Everyday Favorites, Chicken Fettuccini	6	3	0
Stouffer's Turkey Tetrazzini	18	7	-
Swanson American Recipes, Chicken Strips	28	6	+
Swanson American Recipes, Classic Fried Chicken	36	8	-
Swanson American Recipes, Grilled Turkey Medallions	14	3.5	-
Swanson American Recipes, Stuffed Baked Turkey	11	3	-
Swanson Hungry Man, Beer Battered Chicken & Cheese Fries	26	10	+
Swanson Hungry Man, Buffalo Style Chicken Strips	28	6	+
Swanson Hungry Man, Classic Fried Chicken	40	10	+
Swanson Hungry Man, Grilled Smothered Chicken	24	8	+
Swanson Hungry Man, Turkey Breast	22	5	-
Tyson Breast Tenderloins	7	1.5	-
Tyson Nuggets	14	3.5	+
Weight Watchers Smart Ones, Chicken Mirabella	2	0.5	0
Weight Watchers Smart Ones, Glazed Chicken	2.5	1.5	0

FROZEN FOODS—DINNERS, ENTRÉES, SIDES *(cont.)*

Food Item	Total Fat	Sat. Fat	Trans Fat
Weight Watchers Smart Ones, Roast Turkey Medallions	2	0.5	-

BEST BETS: Budget Gourmet Orange Glazed Chicken; Cascadian Farms Orange Dijon Chicken; Weight Watchers Smart Ones, Chicken Mirabella; Weight Watchers Smart Ones, Glazed Chicken

Fish

Food Item	Total Fat	Sat. Fat	Trans Fat
Banquet Fish Stick Meal	20	3.5	-
Gorton's Crunchy Breaded Fish Fillets, Lemon Herb	13	2	+
Gorton's Popcorn Fish	20	2.5	+
Gorton's Popcorn Shrimp	12	2	+
Gorton's Tenders, Original	15	2.5	+
Seapack Clam Strips	14	2	0
Seapack Coconut Shrimp	14	13	+
Seapack Jumbo Butterfly Shrimp	9	1	-
Seapack Popcorn Shrimp	11	2	+
Seapack Shrimp Scampi	32	5	-
Stouffer's Tuna Noodle Casserole	16	5	+
Van de Kamp's Breaded Fish Fillets	3	0.5	-
Van de Kamp's Butterfly Shrimp	15	2.5	+
Van de Kamp's Crispy Tenders	14	2.5	+
Van de Kamp's Crunchy Fish Sticks	13	2.5	+
Weight Watchers Smart Ones, Tuna Noodle Gratin	7	2.5	-

BEST BETS: None. See the Baked Breaded Fish Fillets recipe in chapter 6.

FROZEN FOODS—DINNERS, ENTRÉES, SIDES *(cont.)*

Food Item	Total Fat	Sat. Fat	Trans Fat
Mexican			
Amy's Burrito, Beans & Rice, Organic	6	0.5	0
Amy's Burrito, Beans, Rice & Cheese, Organic	1	0	0
Amy's Burrito, Roasted Vegetable & Cheese, Organic	8	1	0
Amy's Enchilada w/Black Beans & Vegetables	5	0.5	0
Amy's Enchilada, Cheese	12	6	0
Amy's Enchilada w/Rice & Beans	8	1	0
Amy's Santa Fe Enchilada Bowl	9	2	0
Banquet Mexican Style Enchilada Combo	12	5	-
Cedar Lane Three Cheese Quesadillas	11	6	0
Cedar Lane Three Layer Enchilada Pie	7	3	0
Cedar Lane Vegetable Enchilada, Low Fat	3	1.5	0
Jose Ole Mexi-Minis, Beef & Cheese Mini Tacos	10	3.5	+
Jose Ole Mexi-Minis, Chicken & Cheese Mini Burritos	3.5	1.5	+
Jose Ole Tacquitos, Beef & Cheese	7	2	+
Jose Ole Tacquitos Chicken & Cheese	8	2	+
Jose Ole Tacquitos, Shredded Beef	2	0	+

FROZEN FOODS—DINNERS, ENTRÉES, SIDES *(cont.)*

Food Item	Total Fat	Sat. Fat	Trans Fat
Patio Beef Tamales & Enchilada Dinner	19	6	-
Patio Beef Taquitos	22	6	0
Stouffer's Chicken Enchiladas, Family Style	14	7	-
Swanson Hungry Man, Mexican Style	33	9	+
Weight Watchers Smart Ones, Chicken Enchiladas Suiza	8	4	-
Weight Watchers Smart Ones, Santa Fe Rice & Beans	8	4	0

BEST BETS: Amy's Burrito, Beans, Rice & Cheese; Cedar Lane Vegetable Enchilada, Low Fat. Also try the Potato Enchilada recipe in chapter 6.

Pasta/Italian

Food Item	Total Fat	Sat. Fat	Trans Fat
Amy's Stuffed Pasta Shells Bowl	12	7	0
Banquet Lasagna w/Meat Sauce, family size	9	3	-
Banquet Lasagna w/Meat Sauce, Value Menu	10	4	-
Banquet Salisbury Steak w/Gravy, family size	18	8	-
Budget Gourmet Classic, Lasagna Alfredo	10	5	-
Budget Gourmet Classic, Macaroni & Cheese	13	6	-

FROZEN FOODS—DINNERS, ENTRÉES, SIDES *(cont.)*

Food Item	Total Fat	Sat. Fat	Trans Fat
Budget Gourmet Classic, Rigatoni w/Cream Sauce w/Broccoli	4	1.5	-
Budget Gourmet Classic, Spaghetti w/Marinara	5	1	-
Budget Gourmet Classic, Ziti Parmesano	7	2.5	-
Budget Gourmet Premium, Cheese Manicotti w/Marinara	13	5	-
Budget Gourmet Premium, Fettuccini & Meatballs	5	1.5	-
Budget Gourmet Premium, Three Cheese Lasagna	14	7	-
Cascadian Farm Pasta Primavera	8	2.5	0
Cascadian Farm Spinach Lasagna	10	6	0
Cedar Lane Cheese Lasagna	12	6	0
Cedar Lane Eggplant Parmesan	8	3	0
Healthy Choice Manicotti, Familiar Favorites	5	3	0
Michael Angelo's Eggplant Parmesan	19	3	0
Michael Angelo's Fettuccine Alfredo	18	8	0
Michael Angelo's Spinach Ravioli	20	9	0
Michael Angelo's Vegetable Lasagna	7	3	0
Michelina's Fettuccine Alfredo	13	7	-
Michelina's Fettuccine Alfredo w/Chicken & Broccoli	11	6	-
Michelina's Homestyle Bowls, Cheese Stuffed Rigatoni	9	5	-
Michelina's Lasagna w/Meat	7	3	-

FROZEN FOODS—DINNERS, ENTRÉES, SIDES *(cont.)*

Food Item	Total Fat	Sat. Fat	Trans Fat
Michelina's Lasagna w/Meat Sauce & Four Cheeses	8	3.5	0
Michelina's Macaroni & Cheese	11	6	-
Michelina's Noodles w/Chicken, Peas & Carrots	10	4.5	-
Michelina's Spaghetti & Meatballs	8	3	-
Michelina's Stuffed Cheese Rigatoni	8	4.5	-
OnCor Lasagna w/Meat Sauce	8	3.5	0
OnCor Mostaccioli w/Meatballs	8	3	0
Stouffer's Italian Sausage Stuffed Rigatoni	16	9	0
Stouffer's Lasagna w/Meat Sauce, Family Style	12	7	-
Stouffer's Lean Cuisine Everyday Favorites, Lasagna w/Meat Sauce	8	4	-
Stouffer's Lean Cuisine Everyday Favorites, Spaghetti	5	1.5	0
Stouffer's Macaroni & Cheese	15	7	-
Stouffer's Macaroni & Cheese, Family Style	18	8	-
Stouffer's Rigatoni w/Roasted Chicken	16	5	0
Stouffer's Vegetable Lasagna, Family Style	18	7	-
Weight Watchers Smart Ones, Three Cheese Zita Marinara	7	2	0

BEST BETS: Stouffer's Lean Cuisine Everyday Favorites, Spaghetti. Also try the Macaroni, Tuna, and Mushroom recipe in chapter 6 and the Garlic Lentil Red Sauce over your favorite pasta.

FROZEN FOODS—DINNERS, ENTRÉES, SIDES *(cont.)*

Food Item	Total Fat	Sat. Fat	Trans Fat
Pizza			
Amy's Cheese Pizza	12	4	0
Amy's Pesto Pizza	12	3.5	0
Amy's Roasted Vegetable Pizza	8	1.5	0
Banquet French Bread Pizza, Pepperoni	18	6	+
Celeste Supreme Pizza	15	6	+
DiGiorno Cheese Stuffed Crust, Four Cheese	14	8	0
DiGiorno Cheese Stuffed Crust, Pepperoni	19	9	0
DiGiorno Cheese Stuffed Crust, Supreme	14	7	0
DiGiorno Deep Dish, Four Cheese	18	9	-
DiGiorno Deep Dish, Pepperoni	22	9	-
DiGiorno Deep Dish, Supreme	17	7	-
DiGiorno Half & Half, Pepperoni & Cheese	18	8	0
DiGiorno Pizza, Four Cheese	9	4.5	0
DiGiorno Pizza, Pepperoni	13	6	-
DiGiorno Pizza, Spinach, Mushroom & Garlic	8	3.5	-
Freschetta Brick Oven Pizza, Classic Supreme	17	7	0
Freschetta Brick Oven Pizza, Five Italian Cheese	14	7	0
Freschetta Brick Oven Pizza, Three Cheese & Bacon	14	6	0

FROZEN FOODS—DINNERS, ENTRÉES, SIDES *(cont.)*

Food Item	Total Fat	Sat. Fat	Trans Fat
Freschetta Four Cheese Pizza	16	8	-
Freschetta Pepperoni Pizza	21	9	-
Freschetta Sauce Stuffed, Pepperoni	16	6	-
Freschetta Special Deluxe	16	7	-
Jeno's Crisp 'N Tasty Pizza Combination	26	6	-
Michelina's Pepperoni Pizza	24	9	-
Red Baron Classic, Mexican Style	19	9	-
Red Baron Classic, Special Deluxe	17	6	-
Red Baron Classic, Supreme	17	7	-
Red Baron Deep Dish, Four Cheese	17	7	-
Red Baron Deep Dish, Meat Trio	20	7	-
Red Baron Deep Dish, Pepperoni	21	7	-
Red Baron Deep Dish, Supreme	21	7	-
Red Baron Pizzeria Style, Four Cheese	13	6	-
Red Baron Pizzeria Style, Pepperoni	18	6	-
Red Baron Pizzeria Style, Special Deluxe	17	6	-
Tombstone Bacon Cheeseburger Pizza	20	9	-
Tombstone BBQ Chicken Pizza	12	6	-
Tombstone Original, 4 Cheese	20	9	-
Tombstone Original, Extra Cheese	15	7	-
Tombstone Original, Pepperoni	18	8	-
Tombstone Original, Pepperoni & Sausage	18	8	-

FROZEN FOODS—DINNERS, ENTRÉES, SIDES *(cont.)*

Food Item	Total Fat	Sat. Fat	Trans Fat
Tombstone Original, Supreme	14	6	-
Totino's Crisp Party Pizza, Cheese	14	5	+
Totino's Crisp Party Pizza, Combo	21	5	+
Totino's Crisp Party Pizza, Pepperoni	21	5	+
Totino's Crisp Party Pizza, Sausage	20	4.5	+

BEST BET: Amy's Roasted Vegetable Pizza. Also try the Pizza recipe in chapter 6.

Pot Pies

Food Item	Total Fat	Sat. Fat	Trans Fat
Banquet Beef Pot Pie	23	11	-
Banquet Chicken Pot Pie	22	9	-
Claim Jumper Beef Pot Pie	41	9	+
Claim Jumper Chicken Pot Pie	39	11	+
Claim Jumper Chicken & Broccoli Pot Pie	38	11	+
Marie Callender's Chicken Pot Pie	38	10	+
Swanson Beef Pot Pie	21	8	+
Swanson Chicken Pot Pie	23	10	+
Swanson Turkey Pot Pie	20	7	+
Swanson Hungry Man Chicken Pot Pie	29	10	+

BEST BETS: None. Try the Pot Pie recipe in chapter 6.

Sandwiches/Pockets

Food Item	Total Fat	Sat. Fat	Trans Fat
Amy's Pocket Sandwich, Cheese Pizza	9	3.5	0

FROZEN FOODS—DINNERS, ENTRÉES, SIDES *(cont.)*

Food Item	Total Fat	Sat. Fat	Trans Fat
Amy's Pocket Sandwich, Roasted Vegetable	8	1.5	0
Amy's Pocket Sandwich, Spinach Feta	9	4.5	0
Amy's Pocket Sandwich, Vegetable Pie	9	1.5	0
Croissant Pockets, Five Cheese Pizza	20	8	-
Croissant Pockets, Ham & Cheese	16	6	-
Croissant Pockets, Meatballs & Mozzarella	14	5	-
Croissant Pockets, Pepperoni Pizza	19	8	-
Hot Pockets, Three Cheese & Chicken Quesadilla	10	4	-
Hot Pockets, Four Meat & Four Cheese Pizza	19	9	0
Hot Pockets, Beef Taco	13	5	-
Hot Pockets, Cheeseburger	14	6	-
Hot Pockets, Ham & Cheese	11	4.5	-
Hot Pockets, Meatballs & Mozzarella	14	5	-
Hot Pockets, Pepperoni Pizza	17	6	-
Hot Pockets, Philly Steak & Cheese	18	7	-
Hot Pockets, Steak Fajita	10	4.5	-
Hot Pockets, Turkey & Ham w/Cheese	13	5	-
Lean Pockets, BBQ	7	2	-
Lean Pockets, Pepperoni Pizza	7	2.5	-
Lean Pockets, Philly Steak & Cheese	7	2.5	-

FROZEN FOODS—DINNERS, ENTRÉES, SIDES *(cont.)*

Food Item	Total Fat	Sat. Fat	Trans Fat
Lean Pockets, Sausage & Pepperoni Pizza	7	2.5	-
Lean Pockets, Turkey Broccoli & Cheese	7	2.5	-
Michelina's Hot Subs, Chicken BBQ	10	4	-
Michelina's Hot Subs, Chicken Caesar	15	6	-
Michelina's Hot Subs, Chicken & Fire Roasted Tomatoes	7	2.5	-
Michelina's Hot Subs, Ham & Cheese	14	7	-
Michelina's Hot Subs, Hot Dog w/Works	21	11	0
Michelina's Hot Subs, Meatball	12	4.5	-
Michelina's Hot Subs, Sloppy Joes	14	6	-
Michelina's Hot Subs, Tuna Melt	8	4	0

BEST BETS: None. Try the Pita Pinto Pockets or Potato Enchiladas recipes in chapter 6.

Sides/Snacks

Food Item	Total Fat	Sat. Fat	Trans Fat
Joseph Hearth Baked Five Cheese Texas Toast	4.5	1	+
Joseph Hearth Baked Garlic Texas Toast	9	2	+
Mama Bella Cheese Garlic Toast	12	3.5	+
Mama Bella Garlic Breadsticks	6	1.5	+
Mama Bella Garlic Toast, Traditional	7	1.5	+

FROZEN FOODS—DINNERS, ENTRÉES, SIDES *(cont.)*

Food Item	Total Fat	Sat. Fat	Trans Fat
Mama Bella Parmesan Cheese Garlic Bread	9	3	+
Ore-Ida Bagel Bites, Cheese & Pepperoni	7	4	0
Ore-Ida Bagel Bites, Cheese, Sausage & Pepperoni	6	3	0
Ore-Ida Bagel Bites, Spicy Nacho	10	3.5	+
Ore-Ida Bagel Bites, Ultra Five Cheese	7	4	0
Pepperidge Farm Texas Toast, Five Cheese	7	2	+
Pepperidge Farm Texas Toast, Garlic	10	1.5	+
Pepperidge Farm Texas Toast, Mozzarella & Monterey Jack	7	1.5	-
T.G.I. Friday's Buffalo Wings	13	3	-
T.G.I. Friday's Chicken Quesadilla Rolls	13	4	-
T.G.I. Friday's Potato Skins, Cheddar & Bacon	11	4.5	+
T.G.I. Friday's Steak Quesadilla Rolls	11	4.5	-

BEST BETS: None. Try the French Baked Potato recipe in chapter 6 and dip them in salsa or a nonrefrigerated dressing from the Best Bets in the "Dips, Dressings and Oils" list.

FROZEN FOODS—VEGETABLES

Note: Virtually all vegetables are fat free when served alone (i.e., without added ingredients); therefore, we have not listed vegetables that were frozen in their natural state. (For fresh and canned vegetables, see "Vegetables, Beans & Soy.") This entry includes frozen vegetables that appear in combination with other foods or have been processed in ways that add fats.

Food Item	Total Fat	Sat. Fat	Trans Fat
Assorted Vegetables			
Green Giant Baby Brussel Sprouts & Butter, box	1	0.5	0 ·
Green Giant Baby Vegetable Medley & Butter, box	1	0.5	0
Green Giant Broccoli & Three Cheese Sauce, bag	2	1	0
Green Giant Cauliflower & Cheese, box	2.5	0.5	+
Green Giant Cauliflower & Three Cheese Sauce, bag	1.5	0.5	0
Green Giant Roasted Potatoes, Broccoli & Cheese, bag	3	1.5	-
Green Giant Create-A-Meal, Stir Fry Lo Mein	1.5	0	-
Green Giant Create-A-Meal, Stir Fry Teriyaki	0.5	0	0
Green Giant Pasta Accents, Alfredo	7	2	-
Green Giant Pasta Accents, Garlic	10	5	-

BEST BETS: All fresh, frozen, or canned vegetables (in that order; canned vegetables often contain a lot of salt unless you buy unsalted varieties) in their natural state. Of the assorted vegetables: Green Giant Baby Brussel Sprouts & Butter, Baby Vegetable Medley & Butter, Broccoli & Three Cheese Sauce, Cauliflower & Three Cheese Sauce, and Create-A-Meal Stir Fry Teriyaki

FROZEN FOODS—VEGETABLES *(cont.)*

Food Item	Total Fat	Sat. Fat	Trans Fat
Potatoes/Onion Rings			
Lamb Weston Long Branch Fries	7	2	+
Lamb Weston Roasted Red Skin Potatoes	2	0	0
Lamb Weston Simply Shreds	0	0	0
Lamb Weston Tasty Qs	9	2	+
Lamb Weston Tater Babies	5	1	+
Lamb Weston Tater Puffs	7	2	+
Mrs. T's Pierogies, Potato & Onion	2	0	-
Ore-Ida Crispers	12	2.5	+
Ore-Ida Fast Food Fries	7	1	+
Ore-Ida Golden Fries	3.5	0.5	+
Ore-Ida Gourmet Onion Rings	10	1.5	+
Ore-Ida Hash Brown Patties	0	0	0
Ore-Ida Potatoes O'Brien	0	0	0
Ore-Ida Steak Fries	3	0.5	+
Ore-Ida Tater Tots	8	1.5	+
Ore-Ida Vidalia O's	15	2.5	+

BEST BETS: Lamb Weston Roasted Red Skin; Lamb Weston Simply Shreds; Ore-Ida Hash Brown Patties; Ore-Ida Potatoes O'Brien. Also try the French Baked Potato and Onion Rings recipes in chapter 6.

FRUIT

Note: Virtually all fresh, dried, and frozen fruits are fat free; therefore, we have not listed them separately. Two exceptions are the avocado, which is high in monounsaturated fat (about 30 grams per fruit), but contains no trans fats. The other is dried banana chips, which contain about 8 grams of fat per ¼ cup serving, but again, no trans fats.

THE TRANS FAT REMEDY

GRAINS

Food Item	Total Fat	Sat. Fat	Trans Fat
Asian Dinners/Noodles			
China Boy Chow Mein Noodles, bag	5	1	+
La Choy Beef Chow Mein, can	1.5	0.5	0
La Choy Beef Pepper Oriental	2	1	0
La Choy Chicken Chow Mein	3	1.5	0
La Choy Chicken Sweet 'N Sour	2	0.5	-
La Choy Chow Mein Noodles, can	6	1	+
Lipton Asian Side Dish, Beef Lo Mein	2.5	0.5	0
Lipton Asian Side Dish, Sweet & Sour Noodles	2	0	0
Lipton Asian Side Dish, Teriyaki Noodles	3	0.5	0

BEST BETS: La Choy Beef Chow Mein; La Choy Beef Pepper Oriental; La Choy Chicken Chow Mein; Lipton Asian Sweet & Sour Noodles; Lipton Asian Teriyaki Noodles

Food Item	Total Fat	Sat. Fat	Trans Fat
Grain Mixes			
Casbah Falafel	3	0	0
Fantastic Falafel	2	0	0
Fantastic Hummus	3	0.5	0
Fantastic Nature's Burger	3	0	0
Near East Couscous, Broccoli & Cheese, prepared	3.5	2	0
Near East Couscous, Herbed Chicken, prepared	3.5	0.5	0

GRAINS *(cont.)*

Food Item	Total Fat	Sat. Fat	Trans Fat
Near East Couscous, Mediterranean Curry, prepared	3.5	0.5	0
Near East Couscous, Plain, prepared	2	0	0
Near East Couscous, Roasted Garlic & Olive Oil, prepared	4.5	0.5	0
Near East Couscous, Toasted Pine Nut, prepared	6	1	0
Near East Taboule, prepared	3	0.5	0

BEST BETS: All except Near East Couscous, Roasted Garlic & Olive Oil and Toasted Pine Nut

Pasta (Canned)

	Total Fat	Sat. Fat	Trans Fat
Chef Boyardee Beefaroni	9	4.5	0
Chef Boyardee Beef Ravioli w/ Tomato & Meat Sauce	7	3	0
Chef Boyardee Cheesy Burger Macaroni	6	2.5	0
Chef Boyardee Cheesy Burger Ravioli	7	3	0
Chef Boyardee Lasagna	10	5	0
Chef Boyardee Overstuffed Beef Ravioli	4.5	2	0
Chef Boyardee, Pepperoni Pizzazoroli	11	3.5	0
Chef Boyardee, Spaghetti & Meatballs w/Tomato Sauce	11	5	0
Franco-American RavioliOs	10	4	-

GRAINS *(cont.)*

Food Item	Total Fat	Sat. Fat	Trans Fat
Franco-American SpaghettiOs, A to Z	1	0.5	0
Franco-American SpaghettiOs w/Calcium	1	0.5	0
Franco-American SpaghettiOs w/Meatballs	8	3.5	-
Franco-American SpaghettiOs, w/Sliced Franks	10	4	-
Franco-American SpaghettiOs w/Tomato Sauce & Cheese	2	1	0

BEST BETS: Franco-American SpaghettiOs, A to Z; Franco-American SpaghettiOs w/Calcium; Franco-American SpaghettiOs w/Tomato Sauce & Cheese

Pasta (Dry)

	Total Fat	Sat. Fat	Trans Fat
American Beauty, all	1	0	0
Barilla, all	1	0	0
Creamette, Healthy Harvest	1.5	0	0
Creamette, regular, all	1	0	0
No Yolks Egg-free noodles	0.5	0	0
Ronzoni, all	1	0	0

BEST BETS: All

Pasta (Mixes)

	Total Fat	Sat. Fat	Trans Fat
Betty Crocker Suddenly Pasta Salad, Classic, prepared	7	1	-

GRAINS *(cont.)*

Food Item	Total Fat	Sat. Fat	Trans Fat
Betty Crocker Suddenly Pasta Salad, Ranch & Bacon, prepared	20	3	+
Chef Boyardee Deep Dish Meals, Cheesy Burger Macaroni	12	4.5	-
Chef Boyardee Deep Dish Meals, Cheese Lover's Lasagna	14	5	-
Chef Boyardee Deep Dish Meals, 5-Cheese Ravioli	13	4.5	-
Chef Boyardee Deep Dish Meals, Pepperoni & Sausage Rotini	9	3	-
Kraft Easy Mac, prepared	8	2.5	+
Kraft Deluxe Four Cheese Macaroni, prepared	10	3.5	0
Kraft Deluxe Macaroni & Cheese Dinner, prepared	10	3.5	0
Kraft Deluxe Rotini & White Cheddar Sauce w/Broccoli, prepared	15	6	0
Kraft Macaroni & Cheese, prepared	18.5	5	0
Kraft Macaroni & Cheese, Spirals, prepared	18.5	5	0
Kraft Macaroni & Cheese, Thick & Creamy, prepared	18.5	5	0
Kraft Macaroni & Cheese, Three Cheeses, prepared	18.5	4.5	0
Kraft Spaghetti Classics, Tangy Italian, prepared	2	0.5	0
Kraft Velveeta Shells & Cheese, prepared	13	4	0

GRAINS (cont.)

Food Item	Total Fat	Sat. Fat	Trans Fat
Lipton Pasta Sides, Chicken, prepared	9	2	-
Lipton Pasta Sides, Chicken & Broccoli, prepared	10.5	3	-
Lipton Pasta Sides, Stroganoff, prepared	10.5	3.5	-
Pasta Roni, Angel Hair Pasta w/Parmesan, prepared	14	4	+
Pasta Roni, Butter & Garlic, prepared	8	2	+
Pasta Roni, Fettuccine Alfredo, prepared	25	6	+
Pasta Roni, Garlic Alfredo, prepared	14	4	+
Pasta Roni, Shells & White Cheddar, prepared	13	3.5	+
Pasta Roni, White Cheddar & Broccoli w/Rigatoni, prepared	14	3.5	+
Pasta Roni Homestyle Deluxe, Creamy Garlic, prepared	17	4.5	+
Pasta Roni Homestyle Deluxe, Four Cheese, prepared	16	4.5	+
Pasta Roni Homestyle Deluxe, Homestyle Chicken, prepared	13	3	+

BEST BET: Kraft Spaghetti Classics, Tangy Italian. Better yet, prepare your favorite dry pasta and serve it with one of the Best Bets in the "Sauces" list (Pasta, Nonrefrigerated).

GRAINS *(cont.)*

Food Item	Total Fat	Sat. Fat	Trans Fat
Rice Mixes			
Knorr Italian Rice, Mushroom Risotto	1	0.5	-
Knorr Italian Rice, Onion Herb Risotto	1.5	0.5	-
Knorr Italian Rice, Risotto Milanese	1	0.5	-
Knorr Pilaf Rice, Chicken	1	0.5	-
Knorr Pilaf Rice, Lemon, Herb, Jasmine Rice	2	1	-
Knorr Pilaf Rice, Original	0.5	0	-
Lipton Rice Side, Asian Teriyaki	1	0	0
Lipton Rice Side, Cheddar Broccoli	2.5	1	-
Lipton Rice Side, Chicken	3	1	-
Lipton Rice Side, Chicken Broccoli	2	0	-
Lipton Rice Side, Mushroom	1	0	-
Lipton Rice Side, Spanish	1	0	-
Lipton Rice & Sauce, Creamy Garlic Parmesan	5	2.5	-
Rice-A-Roni, Beef, prepared	9	2	0
Rice-A-Roni, Broccoli au Gratin, prepared	17	4.5	+
Rice-A-Roni, Chicken, prepared	9	2	0
Rice-A-Roni, Chicken & Broccoli, prepared	5	1	0
Rice-A-Roni, Chicken Teriyaki, prepared	8	1.5	0
Rice-A-Roni, Four Cheese, prepared	12	3	+
Rice-A-Roni, Fried Rice, prepared	11	2	0

GRAINS *(cont.)*

Food Item	Total Fat	Sat. Fat	Trans Fat
Rice-A-Roni, Garden Vegetable, prepared	6	1.5	+
Rice-A-Roni, Mexican Style, prepared	8	1.5	0
Rice-A-Roni, Spanish Rice, prepared	8	1.5	0
Zatarain's New Orleans Style, Chicken Creole	1	0	-
Zatarain's New Orleans Style, Dirty Rice	0	0	-
Zatarain's New Orleans Style, Garlic & Herb	1	0.5	0
Zatarain's New Orleans Style, Jambalaya	0	0	-
Zatarain's New Orleans Style, Red Beans & Rice	0	0	-
Zatarain's New Orleans Style, Spanish	0	0	-

BEST BETS: Lipton Asian Teriyaki; Zatarain's Garlic & Herb

HEALTH & NUTRITION BARS

Food Item	Total Fat	Sat. Fat	Trans Fat
Atkins Advantage Low-Carb Bar, Almond Brownie	8	4	0
Atkins Advantage Low-Carb Bar, Chocolate Coconut	11	8	0

HEALTH & NUTRITION BARS *(cont.)*

Food Item	Total Fat	Sat. Fat	Trans Fat
Atkins Advantage Low-Carb Bar, Chocolate Mocha Crunch	10	6	0
Balance Energy Bar, Almond Brownie	6	1.5	0
Balance Energy Bar, Mocha Chip	6	3.5	0
Balance Energy Bar, Peanut Butter	6	2.5	0
Balance Energy Bar, Yogurt Berry	6	3	0
Balance Energy Bar, Yogurt Honey Peanut	6	3	0
Clif Luna Bar, Cherry Covered Chocolate	4	3	0
Clif Luna Bar, Chcolate Pecan Pie	4.5	3	0
Clif Luna Bar, Key Lime Pie	4	3	0
Clif Luna Bar, LemonZest	4	3	0
Clif Luna Bar, Nuts Over Chocolate	4.5	2.5	0
Clif Luna Bar, Orange Bliss	4	3	0
GeniSoy Protein Bar, Café Mocha Fudge	4	2.5	0
GeniSoy Protein Bar, Chunky Peanut Butter Fudge	7	2.5	0
GeniSoy Protein Bar, Fudge Cookies & Cream	4.5	2.5	0
PowerBar Harvest, Banana Nut	5	2	0
PowerBar Harvest, Carrot Cake	5	2	0
PowerBar Harvest, Iced Oatmeal Raisin	5	2	0
PowerBar Harvest, Toffee Chocolate Chip	5	2	0

HEALTH & NUTRITION BARS *(cont.)*

Food Item	Total Fat	Sat. Fat	Trans Fat
PowerBar Performance, Cappuccino	2	0.5	0
PowerBar Performance, Chocolate	2	0.5	0
PowerBar Performance, Cookies & Cream	3.5	0.5	0
PowerBar Performance, Oatmeal Raisin	2.5	0.5	0
PowerBar Performance, Peanut Butter	3.5	0.5	0
PowerBar Performance, Vanilla Crisp	2.5	0.5	0
PowerBar Pria, Chocolate Honey Graham	3	2	0
PowerBar Pria, Chocolate Peanut Crunch	3	2.5	0
PowerBar Pria, French Vanilla Crisp	3	2.5	0
PowerBar Pria, Strawberry Shortcake	3	2.5	0
PowerBar ProteinPlus, Chocolate Fudge Brownie	5	3	0
PowerBar ProteinPlus, Chocolate Peanut Butter	5	2.5	0
PowerBar ProteinPlus, Cookies & Cream	5	3.5	0
PowerBar ProteinPlus, Vanilla Yogurt	5	3.5	0

BEST BETS: PowerBar—all; PowerBar Pria, Chocolate Honey Graham

MARGARINE, SPREADS & BUTTER

Food Item	Total Fat	Sat. Fat	Trans Fat
Margarine/Spreads			
Benecol	9	1	-
Benecol, Light	5	0.5	-
Blue Bonnet, stick	9	2	+
Blue Bonnet, Light, tub	4.5	1	+
Brummel & Brown, tub (says "no trans fat" on label)	5	1	-
Canola Harvest, tub	11	1.5	+
Country Crock, stick	8	1.5	+
Country Crock, tub	7	1.5	+
Country Crock, Light, tub	5	1	+
Country Crock, tub, with calcium	5	1	-
Country Crock, tub, with yogurt	4.5	1	+
Country Crock, whipped, squeeze	7	1	-
Fleischmann's, Original, stick	11	2	+
Fleischmann's, Original, tub	9	1.5	+
Fleischmann's, Olive oil, tub	8	1.5	+
I Can't Believe It's Not Butter, stick	10	2	+
I Can't Believe It's Not Butter, spray, all flavors	0	0	0
I Can't Believe It's Not Butter, tub	10	2	+
I Can't Believe It's Not Butter, Light, tub	5	1	+
I Can't Believe It's Not Butter, whipped, squeeze	7	4	-
Nucoa	11	2	+
Parkay, stick	10	2	+
Parkay, squeeze	8	1.5	-

MARGARINE, SPREADS & BUTTER *(cont.)*

Food Item	Total Fat	Sat. Fat	Trans Fat
Parkay, tub	8	1.5	+
Promise, tub (contains partially hydrogenated oil, yet no trans fats)	8	2	-
Promise, Fat Free, tub	0	0	0
Smart Balance Plus, tub	9	2.5	0
Smart Balance, squeeze (nonmargarine)	0	0	0
Smart Balance, Light, tub	5	1.5	0
Take Control, Light	5	0.5	0

BEST BETS: I Can't Believe It's Not Butter spray, all flavors; Promise tub, Fat Free; Smart Balance, squeeze

Butter

Challenge Butter	11	7	0
Challenge Butter, European	12	8	0
Land O' Lakes Butter	11	8	0
Land O' Lakes Butter, Soft Baking, with Canola	11	5	0

BEST BETS: None. Use one of the Best Bets under "Margarines," or olive oil (as a bread spread).

MEAT, FISH & POULTRY

Note: Information on fresh meat, poultry, and fish is from United States Department of Agriculture statistics.

MEAT, FISH & POULTRY (cont.)

Food Item	Total Fat	Sat. Fat	Trans Fat
Fish/Shellfish (Fresh)			
Bass, striped, prepared w/o fat, 3.5 ounces	2.3	0.5	0
Clams, raw, 3 ounces	1	0	0
Cod, prepared w/o fat, 3 ounces	1	0	0
Flounder, baked w/o fat, 3 ounces	1	0	0
Haddock, prepared w/o fat, 3 ounces	1	0	0
Halibut, baked w/o fat, 3 ounces	2	0	0
Lobster, steamed and prepared w/o fat, 3 ounces	1	0	0
Mackerel, prepared w/o fat, 3 ounces	15	4	0
Oysters, raw, 8 ounces	6	2	0
Salmon, coho, prepared w/o fat, 3 ounces	6	1	0
Salmon, red, baked w/o fat, 3 ounces	9	2	0
Scallops, steamed and prepared w/o fat, 3 ounces	1	0.5	0
Shrimp, prepared w/o fat, 3 ounces	1	0	0
Snapper, prepared w/o fat, 3 ounces	1	0	0
Sole, baked w/o fat, 3 ounces	1	0	0
Trout, baked w/o fat, 3 ounces	6	2	0
Tuna steak, baked w/o fat, 3 ounces	1	0	0

BEST BETS: All except mackerel, oysters, and tuna steak. Although tuna steak meets our criteria, it is high in mercury and thus we can't recommend it as a Best Bet. Salmon doesn't meet our Best Bet criteria, but it is regarded as a healthy fish and so we have included it. Note, however, that farmed salmon (more than 60 percent of salmon sold in the U.S. is farmed) contains less healthy fats and more pesticide residues than wild salmon and therefore is not recommended.

MEAT, FISH & POULTRY *(cont.)*

Food Item	Total Fat	Sat. Fat	Trans Fat
Fish (Processed)			
Chicken of the Sea Albacore Tuna, in water	4	2	0
Chicken of the Sea Pink Salmon	2	1	0
StarKist Albacore Tuna, in water	1	0	0

BEST BETS: All; however, pregnant women and young children should limit their intake of tuna, especially albacore, because of its mercury content. Young children should not eat more than one 6-ounce can of albacore tuna every 3 to 4 weeks; pregnant women, one can every 6 to 12 days.

Meat (Fresh)			
Beef, chuck, arm pot roast, lean only, 3 ounces	9	3	0
Beef, chuck, arm pot roast, lean & fat, 3 ounces	22	9	0
Beef, chuck, blade roast, lean only, 3 ounces	13	6	0
Beef, chuck, blade roast, lean & fat, 3 ounces	26	11	0
Beef, flank, broiled, 3 ounces	13	5	0
Beef, ground, panfried, regular, 3 ounces	16	6	0
Beef, ground, panfried, lean, 3 ounces	15	6	0
Beef, T-bone steak, lean only, 3 ounces	9	4	0

MEAT, FISH & POULTRY (cont.)

Food Item	Total Fat	Sat. Fat	Trans Fat
Beef, T-bone steak, lean & fat, 3 ounces	21	9	0
Beef, tenderloin steak, 3 ounces	10	4	0
Beef, top round steak, 3 ounces	5	2	0
Ham, cured, extra lean, 3 ounces	5	2	0
Ham, cured, regular, 3 ounces	8	3	0
Ham, fresh, roasted, lean & fat, 3 ounces	18	6	0
Lamb, rib, roasted, lean only, 2 ounces	7	3	0
Lamb, rib, roasted, lean & fat, 3 ounces	26	12	0
Lamb chop, arm, braised, lean only, 1.7 ounces	7	3	0
Lamb chop, arm, braised, lean & fat, 2.2 ounces	15	7	0
Lamb chop, loin, broiled, lean only, 2.3 ounces	6	3	0
Lamb chop, loin, broiled, lean & fat, 2.8 ounces	16	7	0
Lamb leg, roasted, lean only, 2.6 ounces	6	2	0
Lamb leg, roasted, lean & fat, 3 ounces	13	6	0
Pork, bacon, 3 ounces	42	15	0
Pork, chops, broiled, center loin, 3 ounces	9	3	0
Pork, chops, broiled, center rib, 3 ounces	13	4	0

MEAT, FISH & POULTRY *(cont.)*

Food Item	Total Fat	Sat. Fat	Trans Fat
Pork, fresh rib, roasted, lean & fat, 3 ounces	20	7	0
Pork, sausage, fresh, 3 ounces	26	9	0
Pork, shoulder, braised, lean & fat, 3 ounces	22	8	0
Pork, spareribs, 3 ounces	26	10	0

BEST BETS: Both the top round beef steak and cured ham (extra lean) have slightly higher total fat contents than our criteria, but we included them as Best Bets anyway. Alternatives include the vegetarian "meats" below.

Meat (Processed)

Food Item	Total Fat	Sat. Fat	Trans Fat
Armour Luncheon Meat, can	16	6	0
Dinty Moore Beef Stew, can	8	3.5	0
Hormel Beef Tamales, can	10	4	0
Hormel Corned Beef, can	7	3	0
Hormel Chunk Lean Ham, can	6	2.5	0
Hormel, Mary Kitchen Corned Beef Hash, 50% Reduced Fat, can	12	5	0
Hormel, Mary Kitchen Corned Beef Hash, can	24	11	0
Hormel, Mary Kitchen Roast Beef Hash, can	24	10	0
Hormel Roast Beef, can	4	2	0
Johnsonville Beer 'n Bratwurst	25	9	0
Johnsonville Brats, Original	25	9	0

MEAT, FISH & POULTRY *(cont.)*

Food Item	Total Fat	Sat. Fat	Trans Fat
Johnsonville Hot Italian Sausage	25	9	0
Johnsonville Italian Sausage, Mild	25	9	0
Oscar Mayer Bacon, Ready to Serve	5	2	0
Spam	16	6	0
Underwood Deviled Ham Spread	12	3.5	0
Underwood Liverwurst Spread	14	5	0

BEST BET: Hormel Roast Beef, can

Meat (Processed/Deli/Refrigerated)

	Total Fat	Sat. Fat	Trans Fat
Ball Park Franks, Beef	16	7	0
Ball Park Franks, Beef & Pork	16	6	0
Ball Park Franks, Beef, Fat Free	0	0	0
Ball Park Smoked Sausage, Hot & Spicy	17	6	0
Ball Park Smoked Sausage, Pork, Turkey & Beef	17	6	0
Bar-S Bacon	7	2.5	0
Bar-S Deli Ham, Extra Lean, Honey Cured, 96% Fat Free	1.5	0.5	0
Bar-S Deli Ham, Extra Lean, 96% Fat Free	1	0	0
Bar-S Franks, Beef, Jumbo	18	6	0
Bar-S Franks, Chicken, Jumbo	12	3.5	0
Bar-S Franks, Chicken, Pork, & Beef	15	4.5	0
Bar-S Franks, Turkey, Jumbo	9	3	0
Bar-S Polish Sausage	18	5	0

MEAT, FISH & POULTRY *(cont.)*

Food Item	Total Fat	Sat. Fat	Trans Fat
Bar-S Smoked Sausage	18	5	0
Hebrew National Beef Franks	14	6	0
Hebrew National Beef Franks, 97% Fat Free	1.5	1	0
Hebrew National Beef Franks, Reduced Fat	10	4.5	0
Hebrew National Beef Knockwurst	24	10	0
Hebrew National Beef Polish Sausage	21	10	0
Hebrew National Beef Dinner Franks	32	15	0
Nathan's Beef Franks	15	6	0
Oscar Mayer Bacon	6	2	0
Oscar Mayer Beef Franks	13	6	0
Oscar Mayer Beef Franks, Jumbo	17	7	0
Oscar Mayer Cheese Dogs	13	4.5	0
Oscar Mayer Fat Free Wieners	0	0	0
Oscar Mayer XXL Deli Style Franks	22	9	0

BEST BETS: Ball Park Beef Franks, Fat Free; Bar-S Deli Ham, Extra Lean, 96% Fat Free; Hebrew National Beef Franks, 97% Fat Free; Oscar Mayer Fat Free Wieners

Meat (Vegetarian)

Food Item	Total Fat	Sat. Fat	Trans Fat
Bob's Red Mill Texturized Vegetable Protein	0	0	0
Lightlife Smart Dogs	0	0	0
Lightlife Smart Ground, Taco & Burrito, refrigerated	0	0	0

MEAT, FISH & POULTRY *(cont.)*

Food Item	Total Fat	Sat. Fat	Trans Fat
Loma Linda Meatless Redi-Burger, can	2.5	0.5	0
Loma Linda Meatless Tender Bits, can	4.5	0.5	0
Veggie Patch BBQ Riblets	7	1	0
Veggie Patch Buffalo Wings	4	0.5	0
Veggie Patch Veggie Meatballs	6	1	0
Veggie Patch Wow It's Not Beef	0	0	0
Yves Veggie Bologna Deli Slices, refrigerated	1	0	0
Yves Veggie Turkey Deli Slices, refrigerated	2	0	0

BEST BETS: All *except* Loma Linda Meatless Tender Bits, Veggie Patch Meatballs, and Veggie Patch BBQ Riblets

Poultry (Fresh)

	Total Fat	Sat. Fat	Trans Fat
Chicken, fried, with skin, 3 ounces	13	3	0
Chicken, roasted, with skin, 3 ounces	12	2	0
Chicken, roasted, no skin, breast, 3 ounces	3	1	0
Chicken, roasted, no skin, drumstick, 1.6 ounces	2	1	0
Chicken, roasted, no skin, thigh, 3 ounces	9	3	0
Duck, roasted, flesh only, ½ duck	25	9	0
Turkey, roasted, no skin, breast	1	0	0
Turkey, roasted, no skin, leg	3	1	0

BEST BETS: Turkey, roasted, no skin, breast; chicken, roasted, drumstick

MEAT, FISH & POULTRY *(cont.)*

Food Item	Total Fat	Sat. Fat	Trans Fat
Poultry (Processed)			
Dinty Moore Chicken & Dumplings, can	8	2.5	0
Dinty Moore Turkey Stew, can	8	3.5	0
Hormel Chunk Breast of Chicken, can	1	0	0
Hormel Chunk Chicken, can	2.5	1	0
Hormel Chunk Turkey, can	3	1	0
Swanson Chicken & Dumplings, can	13	5	-
Swanson Chicken à la King, can	23	7	0
Underwood Chicken Spread	7	2.5	0

BEST BET: Hormel Chunk Breast of Chicken, can

Food Item	Total Fat	Sat. Fat	Trans Fat
Poultry (Vegetarian)			
Lightlife Chick 'N Strips, refrigerated	0	0	0
Veggie Patch Chicken 'N Veggie Nuggets	7	1	0
Veggie Patch Wow It's Not Chicken	0.5	0	0

BEST BETS: Lightlife Chick 'N Strips; Veggie Patch Wow It's Not Chicken

REFRIGERATED BISCUITS, COOKIES & SWEET ROLLS

Food Item	Total Fat	Sat. Fat	Trans Fat
Biscuits			
Pillsbury Breadsticks, Garlic w/Herbs	6	1.5	+
Pillsbury Breadsticks, Soft	2.5	0.5	+

REFRIGERATED BISCUITS, COOKIES, ROLLS *(cont.)*

Food Item	Total Fat	Sat. Fat	Trans Fat
Pillsbury Crescent Dinner Rolls	6	2	+
Pillsbury Crusty French Loaf	2	0.5	-
Pillsbury Grands! Biscuits	10	2.5	+
Pillsbury Grands! Buttermilk Biscuits	6	1.5	+
Pillsbury Grands! Crescents	15	3.5	+
Pillsbury Grands! Golden Wheat Biscuits, Reduced Fat	7	2	+

BEST BETS: None. Try one of the Best Bets under Bread/Rolls from the "Baked Goods" list or our Anytime Biscuit recipe in chapter 6.

Cookies/Brownies

Nestlé Toll House Chocolate Chips & Fudge	5	1.5	+
Nestlé Toll House Rich Brownies	7	2.5	+
Nestlé Toll House Sugar Cookies	5	1	+
Nestlé Toll House Ultimates, Chocolate Chips & Chunks	11	3	+
Nestlé Toll House Ultimates, Chocolate Chip Lovers	10	3.5	+
Nestlé Toll House Ultimates, Chocolate Chip & Peanut Butter	5	1.5	+
Nestlé Toll House Ultimates, White Chocolate Macadamia Nut	11	5	+
Pillsbury Chocolate Chip Cookies	7	2	+
Pillsbury Double Chocolate Chip & Chunk Cookies	7	2.5	+

REFRIGERATED BISCUITS, COOKIES, ROLLS *(cont.)*

Food Item	Total Fat	Sat. Fat	Trans Fat
Pillsbury Oatmeal Chocolate Chip			
Cookies	6	2	+
Pillsbury Sugar Cookies	5	1.5	+
Pillsbury Ready to Bake Chocolate			
Chunky Chip Cookies	6	2	+
Pillsbury Ready to Bake Chocolate			
Candy Cookies	5	1.5	+
Pillsbury Ready to Bake Peanut			
Butter Cup Cookies	10	3.5	+

BEST BETS: None. Try our Brownie recipe in chapter 6.

Sweet Rolls

Pillsbury Caramel Rolls	7	1.5	+
Pillsbury Cinnamon Rolls	5	1.5	+
Pillsbury Cinnamon Rolls, Reduced			
Fat	3.5	1	+
Pillsbury Grands! Cinnamon Rolls	11	3	+
Pillsbury Grands! Orange Sweet			
Rolls	11	2.5	+

BEST BETS: None. Spread whole fruit jam or honey on a whole-grain roll and heat it in a microwave or toaster oven for a healthier alternative.

SAUCES & GRAVIES

Food Item	Total Fat	Sat. Fat	Trans Fat
Gravy (Can, Jar)			
Boston Market Classic Beef Gravy	1	0.5	-
Franco-American Beef Gravy	1	0.5	0
Franco-American Country Style Cream Gravy	2.5	0.5	+
Franco-American Turkey Gravy	1	0.5	0
Franco-American Slow Roast Classic Beef Gravy	0.5	0	0
Franco-American Slow Roast Classic Chicken Gravy	0.5	0	-
Heinz Classic Chicken Gravy	0	0	-
Heinz Rich Mushroom Gravy	1	0	-
Heinz Roasted Turkey Gravy	1	0	-
Heinz Savory Beef Gravy	1	0	-

BEST BETS: Franco-American Beef Gravy, Turkey Gravy, and Slow Roast Classic Beef Gravy

Food Item	Total Fat	Sat. Fat	Trans Fat
Gravy (Dry Mix)			
Knorr Au Jus	0	0	-
Knorr Hollandaise	0	0	-
Knorr Roasted Pork	0	0	-
McCormick Creamy Garlic Alfredo	6	3.5	-
McCormick Homestyle	1	0	-
McCormick Pesto	0	0	0
McCormick Roasted Chicken & Herb	1	0	0
McCormick Swedish Meatball Seasoning & Sauce	1	0	-

SAUCES & GRAVIES *(cont.)*

Food Item	Total Fat	Sat. Fat	Trans Fat
McCormick Three Cheese Chicken	3	2	0
McCormick Turkey	0	0	0
McCormick Country, Herb Chicken	2	1.5	0
McCormick Country, Low-Fat	2	0.5	+
McCormick Country, Original	3.5	1	+
McCormick Country, Sausage Flavor	3	1	+

BEST BETS: McCormick Pesto, Roasted Chicken & Herb, Three Cheese Chicken, Turkey, and Country Herb Chicken

Pasta Sauce (Nonrefrigerated Jars/Cans)

Food Item	Total Fat	Sat. Fat	Trans Fat
Aunt Penny's White Sauce	6	1	+
Barilla, Italian Cheese	8	2.5	0
Barilla, Mushroom & Garlic	3	0.5	0
Barilla, Sweet Pepper & Garlic	3	0.5	0
Bertolli, Creamy Alfredo	10	5	0
Bertolli, Five Cheese	3	1	0
Bertolli, Marinara	3	0	0
Bertolli, Olive Oil & Garlic	4	0.5	0
Bertolli, Portobello	7	3.5	0
Bertolli, Vidalia Onion with Garlic	2.5	0	0
Classico, Alfredo	6	4	0
Classico, Florentine Spinach & Cheese	4.5	1	0
Classico, Four Cheese	4	1	0
Classico, Garden Vegetable	1	0	-
Classico, Italian Sausage	3	1	0
Classico, Mushroom & Ripe Olive	1	0.5	0

SAUCES & GRAVIES *(cont.)*

Food Item	Total Fat	Sat. Fat	Trans Fat
Classico, Roasted Garlic Alfredo	9	4	0
Classico, Spicy Tomato & Pesto	5	1	0
Classico, Sun Dried Tomato Alfredo	10	4.5	0
Classico, Sweet Basil Marinara	2	0	0
Classico, Tomato & Basil	1	0	0
Classico, Triple Mushroom	2	0.5	-
Emeril's, Roasted Gaaahlic	3	0	0
Emeril's, Roasted Red Pepper	3	0	0
Hunt's, Cheese & Garlic	1	0	0
Hunt's, Garlic & Herb	1	0	0
Hunt's, Roast Garlic & Onion	1	0	0
Newman's Own, Marinara	2	0	0
Newman's Own, Tomato, Peppers & Spices	2	0	0
Newman's Own, Tomato & Roast Garlic	2.5	0	0
Prego, Garden Combination	2	0.5	0
Prego, Italian Sausage & Garlic	5	1.5	0
Prego, Meat Flavor	5	1.5	0
Prego, Mushroom	3.5	1.5	0
Prego, Mushroom Supreme	5	1.5	0
Prego, Roasted Garlic Parmesan	2	0.5	0
Prego, Tomato, Onion & Garlic	3.5	1	0
Prego, Traditional	3	0.5	0
Ragú, Chunky Garden Style, Garden Combination	3	0	0
Ragú, Chunky Garden Style, Super Garden Primavera	3	0	0

SAUCES & GRAVIES *(cont.)*

Food Item	Total Fat	Sat. Fat	Trans Fat
Ragú, Chunky Garden Style, Super Chunky Mushroom	3	0	0
Ragú, Chunky Garden Style, Tomato, Basil & Cheese	3	0	0
Ragú, Chunky Garden Style, Tomato, Garlic & Onion	3	0	0
Ragú, Classic Alfredo	10	3.5	0
Ragú, Old World Style, Meat Flavor	4	1	0
Ragú, Old World Style, Mushroom & Green Pepper	3	0	0
Ragú, Old World Style, Traditional	3	0	0
Ragú, Pizza Quick Snack Sauce	2	0	0
Ragú, Pizza Sauce	1	0	0
Ragú, Rich & Meaty, Classic Italian	10	3	0
Ragú, Rich & Meaty, Mama's Meat Sauce	8	2	0
Ragú, Rich & Meaty, Sausage, Pepper & Onion	11	3.5	0
Ragú, Roasted Garlic Parmesan	10	3	0
Ragú, Robusto, Chopped Tomato, Olive Oil & Garlic	4.5	1.5	0
Ragú, Robusto, Classic Italian Meat	4	1	0
Ragú, Robusto, 7-Herb	3.5	0.5	0
Ragú, Robusto, Six Cheese	3	1	0
Ragú, Robusto, Sweet Italian Sausage & Cheese	4.5	1	0

BEST BETS: With so many good choices, we chose the best of the best: Classico Garden Vegetable; Classico Mushroom and Ripe

Shopping for Your Family

Olive; Classico Tomato & Basil; Classico Triple Mushroom; Hunt's Cheese & Garlic; Hunt's Garlic & Herb; Hunts Roast Garlic & Onion; Newman's Own Marinara; Newman's Own Tomato, Pepper & Spices; Prego Garden Combination; Prego Roasted Garlic Parmesan; Ragú Pizza Quick Snack Sauce; Ragú Pizza Sauce.

Food Item	Total Fat	Sat. Fat	Trans Fat
Salsa/Mexican Sauces			
Arriba! Salsa, all	0	0	0
Clint's Texas Salsa, all	0	0	0
Hatch Creamy Green Chile Cooking Sauce	3	1.5	0
Hatch Green Chile Enchilada Sauce	1	0	0
Hatch Tex-Mex Style Enchilada Sauce	1.5	0	0
Herdez Salsa, all	0	0	0
La Victoria Enchilada Sauce	0	0	0
La Victoria Enchilada Sauce, Green Chile	0	0	0
La Victoria Salsa, all	0	0	0
Newman's Own Salsa, all	0	0	0
Old El Paso Enchilada Sauce	1	0	0
Old El Paso Enchilada Sauce, Green Chile	1.5	0	0
Ortega Salsa, all	0	0	0
Pace Mexican Creations Cooking Sauces, all (except Roasted Ranchero)	0	0	0

SAUCES & GRAVIES *(cont.)*

Food Item	Total Fat	Sat. Fat	Trans Fat
Pace Mexican Creations Cooking Sauce, Roasted Ranchero	1	0	0
Pace Picante and Salsa, all	0	0	0

BEST BETS: All

SNACKS & NUTS

Food Item	Total Fat	Sat. Fat	Trans Fat
Corn/Tortilla chips			
Frito-Lay Corn Chips	10	1.5	0
Frito-Lay Baked Doritos, Nacho Cooler Ranch	3.5	0.5	0
Frito-Lay Doritos, Four Cheese	8	1	-
Frito-Lay Doritos, Ranchero	6	1.5	+
Frito-Lay Doritos, Salsa Verde	7	1	0
Frito-Lay Doritos, Toasted Corn	7	1	0
Frito-Lay Tostitos, Restaurant Style	6	1	0
Frito-Lay Tostitos, Santa Fe	6	1	0
Frito-Lay Tostitos, Scoops	7	1	0
Mission Tortilla Rounds; also Triangles, Strips, Tri-Color	7	3	+

BEST BETS: Frito-Lay Baked Doritos, Nacho Cooler Ranch

Nuts			
Planters Cashews	14	3	-
Planters Dry Roasted Peanuts	13	2	-

SNACKS & NUTS *(cont.)*

Food Item	Total Fat	Sat. Fat	Trans Fat
Planters Mixed Nuts	15	2.5	-
Planters Trail Mix, Fruit & Nuts	7	2	-
Planters Trail Mix, Nuts & Chocolate	11	2.5	-
Planters Trail Mix, Nuts, Cheese Nips & Mini Ritz	12	1.5	-

BEST BETS: None meet our criteria. However, nuts are a good source of protein and can be enjoyed in moderation (1 to 2 ounces) a few times a week; raw, organic nuts are preferred.

Peanut Butter/Nut Spreads

Food Item	Total Fat	Sat. Fat	Trans Fat
Arrowhead Mills Creamy Valencia Peanut Butter	16.5	2.5	0
I.M. Healthy SoyNut Butter, Chocolate	14	2	0
I.M. Healthy SoyNut Butter, Honey Chunky	11	1.5	0
I.M. Healthy SoyNut Butter, Original	11	1.5	0
Jif Peanut Butter, Regular	16	3	+
Jif Peanut Butter, Reduced Fat	12	2.5	+
Kettle Almond Butter, Creamy	16	2	0
Kettle Cashew Butter	14	3	0
Laura Scudders Natural Peanut Butter	16	2	0
Nutella Hazelnut Spread	11	2	-
Peter Pan, Crunchy	16	3.5	+
Peter Pan, Creamy, Reduced Fat	11	2.5	+
Skippy Peanut Butter, Regular	17	3.5	+

SNACKS & NUTS *(cont.)*

Food Item	Total Fat	Sat. Fat	Trans Fat
Skippy Peanut Butter, Reduced Fat	12	2.5	+
Skippy Peanut Butter, squeeze	17	3.5	+
Smucker's Goober Grape (peanut butter & jelly)	13	2	0

BEST BETS: I.M. Healthy SoyNut Butter, Original and Honey Chunky. Although none of the peanut or nut spreads meet our criteria for total fat, several brands have no trans fats and are low in saturated fat, and so we chose the best of the list. Peanut and nut butters are good sources of protein and can be eaten in moderation.

Popcorn

Note: Numbers for all microwave popcorn are for the amount of unpopped product used.

Food Item	Total Fat	Sat. Fat	Trans Fat
Act II Butter, microwave	10	2	+
Act II Classic White, microwave	14	3	+
Act II Kettle Corn, microwave	12	2.5	+
Frito-Lay Smartfood White Cheddar Popcorn, already popped	10	2	0
Gaslamp Kettle Corn, already popped	4.5	0.5	0
Jolly Time Big Cheez, microwave	9	2	+
Jolly Time Blast O Butter, microwave	11	2.5	+
Jolly Time Healthy Pop, Butter Flavor, microwave (says "trans-fat free" but partially hydrogenated oil is second ingredient)	2	0	+

SNACKS & NUTS *(cont.)*

Food Item	Total Fat	Sat. Fat	Trans Fat
Jolly Time Healthy Pop Kettle Corn, microwave	2	0	+
Orville Redenbacher's Butter Light, microwave	5	1	+
Orville Redenbacher's Honey Butter, microwave	12	3	+
Orville Redenbacher's Movie Theater Butter, microwave	12	2.5	+
Orville Redenbacher's Ultimate Butter	11	2.5	+
Pop Secret Butter Jumbo Pop, microwave	12	3	+
Pop Secret Homestyle, microwave	12	2.5	+
Pop Secret Movie Theater Butter, microwave	13	2.5	+
Pop Secret Toffee Butter, microwave	13	3	+
Smart Balance Light Butter Popcorn, microwave	4.5	1.5	0
Smart Balance Movie Palace Popcorn, microwave	11	4	0

BEST BETS: Gaslamp Kettle Corn, Smart Balance Light Butter Popcorn. You can also use a hot air popper to pop your own and add spray-on canola oil along with herbs and spices.

Potato Chips

Food Item	Total Fat	Sat. Fat	Trans Fat
Frito-Lay Baked Potato Chips	1.5	0	0
Frito-Lay Ruffles WOW (w/olestra)	0	0	0
Frito-Lay Ruffles, BBQ	10	2.5	0
Frito-Lay Ruffles, Original	10	3	0

SNACKS & NUTS *(cont.)*

Food Item	Total Fat	Sat. Fat	Trans Fat
Frito-Lay Ruffles, Sour Cream & Onion	10	3	-
Frito-Lay Sun Chips, French Onion	6	0.5	+
Frito-Lay Sun Chips, Original	6	1	0
Poore Brothers Potato Chips, Original; also Salt & Vinegar; also Dill Pickle	9	2.5	0
Poore Brothers Potato Chips, Parmesan & Garlic; also BBQ; also Habanero	9	2.5	0
Pringles, CheezUms	10	3	0
Pringles, Original	11	1.5	0
Pringles, Sour Cream & Onion	10	2.5	-
Pringles, Sweet Mesquite BBG	10	1.5	0

BEST BETS: Frito-Lay Baked Potato Chips; Frito-Lay Ruffles WOW (but these have been known to cause intestinal problems because they contain olestra).

Pretzels

	Total Fat	Sat. Fat	Trans Fat
Frito-Lay Rold Gold, Honey Mustard Tiny Twists	1	0	0
Frito-Lay Rold Gold, Sharp Cheddar Tiny Twists	1	0	-
Snyder's Buttermilk Ranch Pieces	6	1	+
Snyder's Butter Snaps; also Rods, Sticks	1	0	0
Snyder's Garlic Bread Nibblers	3	0.5	+

SNACKS & NUTS *(cont.)*

Food Item	Total Fat	Sat. Fat	Trans Fat
Snyder's Honey Mustard & Onion	7	1	+
Snyder's Jalapeño Pieces	5	1	+
Snyder's Sourdough; also Minis	0	0	0

BEST BETS: Frito-Lay Rold Gold, Honey Mustard Tiny Twists; Snyder's Butter Snaps, Rods, and Sticks; Snyder's Sourdough and Minis

Other

Food Item	Total Fat	Sat. Fat	Trans Fat
Cracker Jacks	2	0	0
Crunch 'n Munch Buttery Toffee Popcorn w/Peanuts	6	1.5	-
Frito-Lay Cheetos, Crunchy	11	1.5	0
Frito-Lay Cheetos, Twisted	10	1.5	-
Frito-Lay Munchies, Classic	6	1	-
Frito-Lay Munchies, Flamin' Hot	6	1	+
Frito-Lay Munchies, Traditional	5	1	-
Frito-Lay Munchies, Ultimate Cheddar	4.5	1	-
Kraft Corn Nuts, BBQ	4.5	0.5	+
Kraft Corn Nuts, Original	4.5	0.5	+
Kraft Corn Nuts, Ranch	5	1	+
Mission Chicharrones, Picante	5	1.5	0
T.G.I. Friday's Potato Skins, Cheddar & Bacon	9	1.5	+
T.G.I. Friday's Potato Skins, Sour Cream & Onion	10	1.5	-

BEST BET: Cracker Jacks

THE TRANS FAT REMEDY

SOUPS

Food Item	Total Fat	Sat. Fat	Trans Fat
Canned			
Campbell's, Bean w/Bacon	4	1.5	0
Campbell's, Cheddar Cheese	5	2.5	+
Campbell's, Cream of Broccoli	3.5	1	0
Campbell's, Cream of Chicken w/Herbs	4	1.5	0
Campbell's, Cream of Potato	3	2	0
Campbell's, Double Noodle	2.5	1	0
Campbell's, Golden Mushroom	3.5	1	-
Campbell's, New England Clam Chowder	2.5	0.5	0
Campbell's, Split Pea w/Ham & Bacon	3.5	2	0
Campbell's, Tomato	1.5	0.5	0
Campbell's, Vegetable w/Beef Stock	0.5	0.5	0
Campbell's, Vegetarian Vegetable	0.5	0	0
Campbell's 98% Fat Free, Cream of Celery	3	1	0
Campbell's 98% Fat Free, Cream of Chicken	2	1	-
Campbell's 98% Fat Free, Cream of Mushroom	3	1	-
Campbell's Chunky, Baked Potato w/Cheddar & Bacon	8	3	-
Campbell's Chunky, Chicken Corn Chowder	13	3	0
Campbell's Chunky, Chicken Dumpling	9	2	-
Campbell's Chunky, Chicken Mushroom Chowder	17	3	0

SOUPS *(cont.)*

Food Item	Total Fat	Sat. Fat	Trans Fat
Campbell's Chunky, Grilled Chicken & Sausage Gumbo	2.5	1	-
Campbell's Chunky, Hearty Bean & Ham	2	1	0
Campbell's Chunky, Hearty Vegetable w/Pasta	3	1	0
Campbell's Chunky, Old Fashioned Potato Ham Chowder	13	5	0
Campbell's Chunky, Old Fashioned Vegetable Beef	2.5	1.5	0
Campbell's Chunky, Sirloin Burger w/Vegetables	8	5	-
Campbell's Chunky, Slow Roasted Beef w/Mushrooms	1.5	1	-
Campbell's Chunky, Tomato Cheese Ravioli w/Vegetables	2.5	1.5	-
Campbell's Healthy Request, Chicken Noodle	2	1	0
Campbell's Healthy Request, Chicken Rice	2	1	0
Campbell's Healthy Request, Cream of Celery	2	1	-
Campbell's Healthy Request, Cream of Chicken	2.5	1	-
Campbell's Healthy Request, Cream of Mushroom	2.5	1	0
Campbell's Kitchen Classics, Bean w/Bacon	4	1.5	0
Campbell's Kitchen Classics, Chicken Noodle	1	0.5	0

SOUPS (cont.)

Food Item	Total Fat	Sat. Fat	Trans Fat
Campbell's Kitchen Classics, Chicken w/White & Wild Rice	1	0.5	0
Campbell's Kitchen Classics, Lentil	0.5	0.5	0
Campbell's Kitchen Classics, Minestrone	0.5	0.5	0
Campbell's Kitchen Classics, New England Clam Chowder	9	2	0
Campbell's Kitchen Classics, Tomato	0	0	0
Campbell's Select, Chicken & Pasta	1	0.5	-
Campbell's Select, Chicken Vegetable	0.5	0	0
Campbell's Select, Creamy Potato	9	2.5	0
Campbell's Select, Grilled Chicken w/Sundried Tomatoes & Mushrooms	1	0.5	0
Campbell's Select, Honey Roasted Chicken w/Potatoes	1	1	0
Campbell's Select, Italian Style Wedding	2.5	2	0
Campbell's Select, New England Clam Chowder, 98% Fat Free	1.5	0.5	0
Campbell's Select, New England Clam Chowder	11	2.5	0
Campbell's Select, Roast Chicken w/Long Grain & Wild Rice	0.5	0	0
Campbell's Select, Tomato Garden	1	0.5	0
Campbell's Soup at Hand, Chicken & Stars	0.5	0.5	0
Campbell's Soup at Hand, Creamy Broccoli	8	2	0

SOUPS *(cont.)*

Food Item	Total Fat	Sat. Fat	Trans Fat
Campbell's Soup at Hand, Mexican Style	2	1	0
Campbell's Soup at Hand, New England Clam Chowder	6	1.5	0
Campbell's Soup at Hand, Pizza	0.5	0.5	0
Campbell's Soup at Hand, Vegetable Medley	2	1.5	0
Healthy Choice, Chicken & Dumplings	3	1	0
Healthy Choice, Chicken Noodle	2	0.5	0
Healthy Choice, Country Vegetable	0.5	0	0
Healthy Choice, Roasted Italian Style Chicken	2	1	0
Healthy Choice, Split Pea & Ham	2.5	1	0
Healthy Valley Fat-Free, Black Bean & Vegetable	0	0	0
Healthy Valley Fat-Free, 5 Bean Vegetable	0	0	0
Healthy Valley Fat-Free, 14 Garden Vegetable	0	0	0
Healthy Valley Fat-Free, Minestrone	0	0	0
Healthy Valley Fat-Free, Tomato Vegetable	0	0	0
Healthy Valley Fat-Free, Vegetable Barley	0	0	0
Healthy Valley Organic, Lentil	2	0	0
Healthy Valley Organic, Potato Leek	2	0	0
Healthy Valley Organic, Split Pea	0	0	0
Pepperidge Farm, Black Bean	2.5	0.5	0
Pepperidge Farm, Chicken w/Wild Rice	3.5	1.5	0
Pepperidge Farm, French Onion	1	0.5	0

SOUPS (cont.)

Food Item	Total Fat	Sat. Fat	Trans Fat
Pepperidge Farm, Gazpacho	2	0.5	0
Pepperidge Farm, Hunters Soup	6	1	0
Pepperidge Farm, Lobster Bisque	11	5	-
Pepperidge Farm, Vichyssoise	8	4.5	0
Progresso, Beef (Steak) & Vegetable	2.5	1.5	0
Progresso, Beef & Baked Potato	2	1	0
Progresso, Chicken Noodle	2	1	0
Progresso, Chicken, Rice w/Vegetables	2	0	0
Progresso, Creamy Tomato	6	2.5	0
Progresso, Grilled Chicken Italiano	2.5	0.5	0
Progresso, Lentil	2	0	0
Progresso, New England Clam Chowder	13	5	+
Progresso, Potato w/Broccoli & Cheese	6	2	-
Progresso, Split Pea	3	1	0
Progresso, Vegetable	1	0	0
Progresso Rich & Hearty, Beef Pot Roast	1.5	0.5	0
Progresso Rich & Hearty, Chicken & Homestyle Noodle	2.5	0.5	0
Progresso Rich & Hearty, Creamy Chicken Wild Rice	5	1.5	-
Progresso Rich & Hearty, Sirloin Steak & Vegetables	1	0	0
Wolfgang Puck, Beef Steak & Potato	6	2.5	0
Wolfgang Puck, Chicken Parmesan w/Pasta	12	5	-
Wolfgang Puck, Chicken w/Sweet Corn	11	4.5	-
Wolfgang Puck, Classic Chicken w/Broccoli	11	1.5	-

SOUPS *(cont.)*

Food Item	Total Fat	Sat. Fat	Trans Fat
Wolfgang Puck, Grilled Chicken w/Rice	5	1.5	0
Wolfgang Puck, Honey Roasted Chicken w/Penne	7	2	-

BEST BETS: These are the best of the best: Campbell's Select: Chicken Vegetable, Grilled Chicken, Roast Chicken w/Long Grain and Wild Rice, and New England Clam Chowder, 98% Fat Free; Campbell's Kitchen Classics: Chicken Noodle, Chicken w/White & Wild Rice, Lentil, Minestrone, Tomato; Campbell's Vegetable w/Beef Stock; Campbell's Vegetarian Vegetable; Campbell's Soup at Hand: Pizza and Chicken & Stars; Healthy Choice Country Vegetable; Healthy Valley Organic: Split Pea and Lentil; Healthy Valley Fat-Free: Vegetable Barley, Black Bean & Vegetable, 5 Bean Vegetable, 14 Garden Vegetable, Minestrone, Tomato Vegetable; Progresso Rich & Hearty Sirloin Steak & Vegetables; Progresso Vegetable

Dry

Food Item	Total Fat	Sat. Fat	Trans Fat
Bear Creek, Cheddar Broccoli	7	2.5	+
Bear Creek, Cheddar Potato Soup Mix	7	2	+
Bear Creek, Creamy Chicken	2	0.5	-
Bear Creek, Creamy Chicken Wild Rice	3.5	1	+
Bear Creek, Creamy Potato Soup Mix	4	1	-
Bear Creek, Navy Bean	4.5	0	-
Bear Creek, Vegetable Beef	0.5	0	0
Fantastic, Big Soup Noodle Bowls, Spring Vegetable	0.5	0	0
Fantastic, Big Soup Noodle Bowls, Vegetarian Beef & Noodles	0	0	0
Fantastic, Big Soup Noodle Bowls, Vegetarian Chicken Noodle	0.5	0	0

SOUPS *(cont.)*

Food Item	Total Fat	Sat. Fat	Trans Fat
Health Valley, Creamy Potato Soup, Fat Free	0	0	0
Health Valley, Chicken Noodle, Fat Free	0	0	0
Health Valley, Corn Chowder, Fat Free	0	0	0
Health Valley, Pasta Parmesan, Fat Free	0	0	0
Knorr, Cream of Spinach	2.5	0.5	-
Knorr, French Onion	1	0.5	-
Knorr, Hot & Sour	1.5	0.5	0
Knorr, Leek	2.5	1	-
Knorr, Spring Vegetable	0	0	-
Knorr, Tomato Beef	2	1	-
Knorr Naturals Hearty Soups, Chunky Potato w/Roast Onions	1	0	0
Knorr Naturals Hearty Soups, Homestyle Chicken Noodle	1.5	0.5	0
Knorr Naturals Hearty Soups, Potato Vegetable	1	0.5	0
Knorr Naturals Hearty Soups, Roast Vegetable w/Long Grain Rice	1	0.5	0
Knorr Savory Soups, Mediterranean Minestrone	2	1	-
Knorr Taste Breaks Soup, Chicken Noodle	1	0	0
Knorr Taste Breaks Soup, Chicken Vegetable	2	0.5	0
Knorr Taste Breaks Soup, Corn Chowder	2.5	0	-

SOUP *(cont.)*

Food Item	Total Fat	Sat. Fat	Trans Fat
Knorr Taste Breaks Soup, Navy Bean	1	0	-
Knorr Taste Breaks Soup, Potato Leek	3.5	0.5	+
Knorr Taste Breaks Soup, Split Pea	0.5	0	0
Lipton Recipe Secrets, Beefy Onion	0.5	0	-
Lipton Recipe Secrets, Extra Noodle	1.5	0.5	0
Lipton Recipe Secrets, Noodle Soup	2	0.5	-
Lipton Recipe Secrets, Onion	0	0	-
Lipton Recipe Secrets, Onion Mushroom	0.5	0	-
Maruchan Instant Lunch, Beef	12	6	+
Maruchan Instant Lunch, Roast Chicken	12	6	+
Maruchan Ramen Noodle Soup, Beef	8	4	+
Maruchan Ramen Noodle Soup, Pork	8	4	+
Maruchan Ramen Noodle Soup, Roast Chicken	8	4	+
Maruchan Ramen Noodle Soup, Shrimp	8	4	+
Mrs. Grass, Noodle	1.5	0.5	-
Mrs. Grass, Onion	0	0	-
Nissin Cup, Noodles Chili Chicken	11	5	+
Nissin Cup, Noodles w/Shrimp	13	7	+

BEST BETS: Bear Creek Vegetable Beef; Fantastic Big Soup Noodle Bowls: Spring Vegetable, Vegetarian Beef & Noodle, Vegetarian Chicken Noodle; Health Valley, all fat free: Creamy Potato, Chicken Noodle, Corn Chowder, Pasta Parmesan; Knorr Taste Breaks: Split Pea

VEGETABLES, BEANS & SOY

Food Item	Total Fat	Sat. Fat	Trans Fat
Beans			
Bush's Baked Beans, BBQ	1	0	0
Bush's Baked Beans, Country Style	1	0	0
Bush's Baked Beans, Maple Cured w/Bacon	1	0.5	0
Bush's Baked Beans, Onion	1.5	0	0
Bush's Baked Beans, Original	1	0	0
Bush's Baked Beans, Vegetarian	0	0	0
Bush's Black Beans	0.5	0	0
Bush's Chili Magic, not prepared	1	0	0
Ranch Style Beans w/Sweet Onions	3	1	-
Ranch Style Blackeye Peas w/Bacon	0.5	0	0
Ranch Style, Original Texas	2.5	1	-
Ranch Style, Pinto w/Jalapeno Peppers	1	0	-
S&W Chili Beans, Zesty Sauce	1	0	0
S&W Chili Makin's, Original	0.5	0	0
S&W Garbanzos	1.5	0	0
S&W Kidney	0.5	0	0
Van Camp's Beanee Weenee	9	3.5	0
Van Camp's Pork & Beans	1.5	0	0

BEST BETS: All *except* Ranch Style Beans w/Sweet Onions, Original Texas, and Pinto w/Jalapeno Peppers; also not Van Camp's Beanee Weenee

Food Item	Total Fat	Sat. Fat	Trans Fat
Chili			
Dennison's, 99% Fat Free, Turkey	3	1	0
Dennison's, Chunky	11	5	0
Dennison's, Hot	15	7	0
Dennison's, Original	13	6	0

VEGETABLES, BEANS & SOY *(cont.)*

Food Item	Total Fat	Sat. Fat	Trans Fat
Hormel Chili, w/Beans	7	3	0
Hormel Chili, Chunky w/Beans	7	3	0
Hormel Chili, Hot, No Beans	9	3	0
Hormel Chili, Turkey w/Beans	3	1	0
Hormel Chili, Vegetarian w/Beans	1	0	0
Stagg Chili, Classic	17	8	0
Stagg Chili, Country Brand	17	7	0
Stagg Chili, Dynamite Hot	17	7	0
Stagg Chili, Fiesta Grill	9	4	0
Stagg Chili, Garden Vegetarian	1	0	0
Stagg Chili, Laredo	15	7	0
Stagg Chili, Ranch House Chicken	11	3	0
Stagg Chili, Rio Blanco Chicken	12	5	0
Stagg Chili, Silverado Beef	3	1	0

BEST BETS: Hormel Chili, Vegetarian w/Beans; Stagg Chili, Garden Vegetarian. Also try the World's Fastest Chili recipe in chapter 6.

Potatoes (Mix)

Food Item	Total Fat	Sat. Fat	Trans Fat
Betty Crocker Potato Buds, not prepared	0	0	0
Betty Crocker Butter & Herb, not prepared	1.5	0	+
Betty Crocker Deluxe Potatoes, Cheesy Cheddar au Gratin, not prepared	4.5	1.5	+
Betty Crocker Deluxe Potatoes, Creamy Roasted Garlic, not prepared	4.5	2	+

VEGETABLES, BEANS, & SOY *(cont.)*

Food Item	Total Fat	Sat. Fat	Trans Fat
Betty Crocker Roasted Garlic Mashed, not prepared	1.5	0	+
Betty Crocker Scalloped, not prepared	1	0	0
Betty Crocker Roasted Garlic Scalloped, not prepared	1.5	0.5	+
Betty Crocker Scalloped, Three Cheese, not prepared	1.5	0.5	+
Hungry Jack, Mashed w/Beef Gravy, prepared	8	2	-
Hungry Jack, Mashed w/Chicken Herb, prepared	8	2	-
Idahoan, Mashed, Butter & Herb, not prepared	2.5	0.5	+
Idahoan, Mashed, Four Cheese, not prepared	2.5	0.5	+
Idahoan, Mashed, Loaded Baked, not prepared	2.5	0.5	+
Idahoan, Mashed, Roasted Garlic, not prepared	2.5	0.5	+

BEST BETS: Betty Crocker Potato Buds; Betty Crocker Scalloped. Also try the French Baked Potato and Stuffed Baked Potato recipes in chapter 6.

Soy/Soybean Products (also see Meat, Vegetarian; and Poultry, Vegetarian)

Food Item	Total Fat	Sat. Fat	Trans Fat
Cabin Ridge Hickory Smoked Tofu	6	1	0
Hinoichi Tofu, Extra Firm	4	0.5	0
Hinoichi Tofu, Firm	3.5	0.5	0
Hinoichi Tofu, Silken Soft	2.5	0	0

VEGETABLES, BEANS, & SOY *(cont.)*

Food Item	Total Fat	Sat. Fat	Trans Fat
Lightlife Gimme Lean Ground Beef Style	0	0	0
Lightlife Gimme Lean Sausage Style	0	0	0
Lightlife Tempeh Garden Vegetable	8	1	0
Soyganic Baked Tofu, Szechuan style	6.6	1	0
Soyrizo	9	0.5	0
Soysage	0.5	0	0

BEST BETS: All Hinoichi tofu; Lightlife Gimme Lean Ground Beef and Sausage; Soysage

Vegetables (Fresh, Canned)
Note: Nearly all fresh and canned vegetables are fat free; all are saturated and trans fat free. Artichokes have about 2 grams of good fat per serving. Corn, green peas, mustard greens, parsnips, and tomatoes have about 1 gram of good fat per serving.

BEST BETS: All

MISCELLANEOUS

Food Item	Total Fat	Sat. Fat	Trans Fat
Packaged Refrigerated Lunches/Snacks			
Armour Lunch Makers, Cracker Crunchers, Cooked Ham	14	7	-
Armour Lunch Makers, Cracker Crunchers, Turkey	14	8	-
Armour Lunch Makers, Pizza, Pepperoni	13	5	-
Funny Bagels, Cheese Pizza	9	5	-
Funny Bagels, Cream Cheese & Jelly	14	8	-
Funny Bagels, Peanut Butter & Jelly	14	3	-

MISCELLANEOUS *(cont.)*

Food Item	Total Fat	Sat. Fat	Trans Fat
Funny Bagels, Turkey & Cheese	13	3.5	0
Oscar Mayer Lunchables Fun Snacks, Oreo Cookies 'n Frosting	8	1.5	+
Oscar Mayer Lunchables Fun Snacks, Fudge Brownies	8	3	+
Oscar Mayer Lunchables, All Star Hot Dogs	19	9	+
Oscar Mayer Lunchables, Cracker Snackers	11	5	-
Oscar Mayer Lunchables, Deep Dish Pizza	15	5	-
Oscar Mayer Lunchables, Fun Fuel Ham Bagels	10	4	0
Oscar Mayer Lunchables, Fun Fuel Turkey Bagels	10	4	0
Oscar Mayer Lunchables, Nachos	29	8	+
Oscar Mayer Lunchables, Pizza, Cheese	15	9	-
Oscar Mayer Lunchables, Pizza, Pepperoni Flavored Sausage	16	8	+
Oscar Mayer Lunchables, Tacos	13	6	-
Oscar Mayer Lunchables, Ultimate Nachos	38	9	+

BEST BETS: None. The high fat, salt, and/or sugar contents in these foods are unhealthy. Healthy lunches for your children can include, for example: any of the Best Bet soups from our list; leftover 30-Minute Gumbo, Pita Pinto Pockets, World's Fastest Chili, Macaroni, Tuna, & Mushrooms, or Vegetable Bean Soup from the recipes in chapter 6; lean turkey slices on whole-grain bread with tomato; peanut butter and banana on whole-grain bread; veggie burger and salsa on whole-grain bun.

CHAPTER 6

What's Cooking?

You've been to the supermarket, so now it's time to create some easy, nutritious meals with all the things you bought. First, let's review what you've learned about trans fats. You now know:

- What trans fats are and the harm they can cause;
- Why trans fats are so popular among food manufacturers;
- How you can decipher Nutrition Facts panels and ingredient lists to uncover the trans fat content of the foods you eat;
- Which foods contain trans fats and approximately how much.

You have enough information to buy and serve your family healthy meals. But we know you are busy, so we would like to help you make nutritious meal preparation much easier. That's why we've provided sample menus for seven days, plus more than two dozen recipes for tasty, virtually trans fat–free and low–saturated fat foods that Americans enjoy the most—from french fries to chili to onion rings to brownies.

Per serving, all of the recipes in this chapter contain no trans fats (less than 0.5 gram) and no more than 2 grams of saturated fat. You'll learn how to take the trans fats out of your food without jeopardizing flavor. You'll discover that this is easier to do than you imagined: Often all it takes is changing one or two ingredients in a traditional recipe—just take a look at our brownie and pizza recipes, for example—or changing how you prepare a particular food.

THREE SQUARES A DAY

Do you depend on frozen waffles or French toast or cereal bars for breakfast? Is your idea of breakfast a fatty sandwich from a fast-food restaurant or a Danish and coffee from the cafeteria? Are your children going to school with prepackaged lunch foods in little trays? Does your lunch come in a paper cup to which you add hot water and stir? Does your dinner come from a drive-up window, or do you reach into the depths of your freezer and pull out a pizza, pot pie, or frozen dinner?

As you saw in chapters 4 and 5, many of these foods are very high in fat, especially trans and saturated fats. What you need are some quick, easy meals you can make at home to take the place of these unhealthy entrées—and in this chapter we give you some of those recipes. You need quick foods that are healthy as well as delicious for active kids. As a bonus, many of the recipes in this chapter freeze well, so you can make a double or triple batch and store the extras in meal-sized packages, ready to pop into the microwave or oven for a fast lunch or dinner the next time you find yourself short on time.

How to Cook and Bake Without Trans Fats

- Instead of frying, sauté, simmer, or stir-fry your vegetables, beans, grains, and fish with vegetable broth, bouillon, soy sauce, wine, or even water flavored with herbs and spices. Once the food is done, you can drizzle in some olive, hempseed, or flaxseed oil for added flavor and healthy monounsaturated fats.
- Steaming is another option. You can use a basket steamer (one that can be placed in any medium- to large-sized pot), a special steamer pot, or a countertop electric steamer. Steaming is an excellent way to prepare vegetables, grains, and fish. Again, you can add a little healthy oil to the finished dish for flavor.
- Crockpots (slow cookers) are invaluable kitchen tools for people on the go or who don't have much time to spend in the kitchen. They allow you to cook foods slowly and gradually so they absorb flavors from the ingredients themselves and any herbs, spices, or other flavorings you add. No oils are needed, but you may want to add a teaspoon or two of olive, hempseed, or flaxseed oil for flavor and healthy fats.
- If you need to fry something, use a minimal

amount of vegetable spray in the bottom of a wok or skillet. Keep stirring the food to prevent sticking.

- Use fat or oil substitutes when baking. Instead of margarine or shortening, you can use unsweetened applesauce, pureed fruit (see box on page 238), or products such as Wonderslim Fat & Egg Substitute.

- Canola oil is another trans fat–free baking substitute for shortening or margarine. Some recipes state that oil can be substituted and will not change the quality of the baked product.

- When baking with fat substitutes, make sure you don't overbake. This is a common error when people first try using fat substitutes for baking. The traditional method of sticking a toothpick or wire cake tester into the center of a cake or muffins doesn't work with fat-free baking. Instead, you need to check doneness by pressing the center of the baked item gently with your finger. If the center springs back, the item is done. You should first check for doneness at the beginning of the time range given in a recipe. That means if it says "Bake for 25 to 35 minutes," make sure you check the cake at 25 minutes; it may be done. Cookies are done when they are just lightly brown around the edges. Even if the centers do not bounce back readily, they will firm up when the cookies cool.

MENUS

Recipes are included for items that are followed by the recipe page number. Some of the recipes that include meat also include a plant-protein alternative (e.g., tofu, TSP) for those who want to avoid or reduce their intake of animal protein.

Day 1

BREAKFAST:
6 ounces tomato juice
Apple Waffles w/applesauce topping (see page 219)
Low-fat milk (regular, soy, or rice milk)

LUNCH:
Pita Pinto Pocket (see page 220)
Fresh fruit
Naturally flavored seltzer

DINNER:
Pasta Wheels w/Garlic Lentil Red Sauce (see page 221)
Tossed salad w/Lite Thousand Island Dressing (see page 222)
Low-fat roll (e.g., sourdough, potato, whole wheat usually have less than 2 grams of saturated fat per serving)
Herbal tea, decaf coffee, or 100% fruit juice

Day 2

BREAKFAST:
6 ounces orange juice
Oatmeal w/raisins and cinnamon
Whole wheat toast w/honey or pure fruit jam
Herbal tea

LUNCH:
Veggie burger (e.g., Boca, Better 'N Burger, Morningstar Spicy Black Bean Burger, Gardenburger Veggie Medley) in whole wheat pita w/tomato and onion slices, ketchup, mustard, relish
French Baked Potatoes (see page 222)
Flavored seltzer

DINNER:
30-Minute Gumbo (see page 223)
Brown rice
Steamed broccoli or zucchini w/salsa
Decaf coffee, herbal tea

Day 3

BREAKFAST:
¼ cantaloupe or ½ grapefruit
Breakfast Muffin (see page 225)
Nonfat yogurt (regular or soy)

LUNCH:
Stuffed Baked Potato (see page 225)
Fresh fruit
Iced herbal tea

DINNER:
World's Fastest Chili (see page 226)
Cucumber and tomato salad w/Garlic Salad Dressing
(see page 227)
Apple Pie (see page 227)
Decaf coffee, low-fat soy or rice milk

Day 4

BREAKFAST:
1 cup whole-grain cereal (e.g., Kashi brand)
½ cup berries
½ whole wheat bagel w/low-fat cream cheese

LUNCH:
World's Fastest Chili leftovers
Fresh fruit

DINNER:
Baked Breaded Fish Fillets (see page 228)
Onion Rings (see page 228)
Steamed broccoli w/drizzled olive oil and herbs

Day 5

BREAKFAST:
Fruit Smoothie (see page 229)
English muffin w/all-fruit jelly
Decaf coffee or tea

LUNCH:
Roasted chicken breast in a whole wheat pita, w/to-
mato, lettuce, and Garlic Salad Dressing (see page 227)
Fresh fruit
Seltzer

DINNER:
MTM: Macaroni, Tuna, and Mushrooms (see page 229)
Tossed salad w/Lite Thousand Island Dressing or Garlic Dressing (see pages 222 or 227)
Brownie (see page 230)

Day 6

BREAKFAST:
Scrambled Black and White (see page 230)
2 soy sausage links (Lightlife; see chapter 5, "Meats, Vegetarian")
1 Anytime Biscuit (see page 231)

LUNCH:
Potato Enchiladas (see page 231)
Fresh fruit
Herbal tea

DINNER:
Pot Pie (see page 232)
String beans sautéed in soy sauce and olive oil
Blueberry Pie (see page 233)

Day 7

BREAKFAST:
Currants and Cornmeal (see page 234)
Sliced cantaloupe or honeydew
Herbal tea

LUNCH:
Vegetable Bean Soup (see page 235)
Whole Wheat Crackers (see page 236)
Herbal tea

DINNER:
Pizza (see page 236)
Tossed salad w/garbanzo beans, olive oil, and vinegar
Decaf coffee or tea

Snacks

Baked, fat-free potato chips or tortilla chips w/salsa
Hot-air popped corn with sprayed-on oil, sprinkled
with salt and herbs
Raisins
Roasted chestnuts
Fresh fruit
Toasted bagel w/natural peanut butter or jelly
No Bake Crispy Bars (see page 237)
Chocolate Pudding (see page 238)

RECIPES

APPLE WAFFLES
Makes about 10 single waffles

2 cups whole wheat flour   *3 Tbs applesauce*
2 tsp baking powder   *2 cups apple juice (or*
2 tsp egg replacer mixed   *water if you prefer a*
* with 4 Tbs water*   *less sweet waffle)*

Use a nonstick waffle iron. Preheat the iron while mix-
ing the ingredients. Combine dry ingredients in a
bowl. Prepare the egg replacer mixture. Combine the
egg replacer mixture, applesauce, and apple juice (or

water) and mix well. Add this mixture to the dry ingredients and stir well. Let the batter stand for 5 minutes until it becomes slightly thick. Ladle batter into the waffle iron and cook waffles for about 5 minutes or until brown. Serve with applesauce or pure maple syrup.

PITA PINTO POCKETS
Makes enough for 3–4 sandwiches

4 ounces ground lean turkey

1 tsp olive oil

1 15-oz can pinto beans, or 1½ cups cooked pinto beans

1 Tbs prepared mustard

1 Tbs tomato paste or ketchup

1 Tbs soy sauce

1 Tbs lemon juice or vinegar

1 tsp onion powder

Whole wheat pita pockets

Tomato slices, lettuce, sprouts, chopped cucumber, or other desired vegetable garnishes

In a nonstick skillet, sauté the ground turkey in a little water and cook until brown. Turn off heat and stir in 1 tsp olive oil. Combine the next six ingredients in a food processor and blend until smooth. If the consistency is too dry, add a few drops of water and stir until desired consistency is reached. Spoon the turkey into each pita pocket, add a layer of the bean mixture, and then top with garnishes.

GARLIC LENTIL RED SAUCE

Makes about 2 cups

2 tsp olive oil
1 medium onion,
  chopped
6 cloves garlic, minced
1 cup water
½ cup dry lentils (or 1
  cup cooked lentils)
½ cup dry red wine
1 28-oz can crushed
  tomatoes

1 Tbs dried oregano
¼ tsp crushed red
  pepper flakes
½ cup fresh basil,
  chopped
Salt and black pepper
  to taste

In a saucepan, heat the oil and add the onion and garlic; cook for about 5 minutes. Add water, dry lentils (skip water and dry lentils if you are using cooked lentils), wine, tomatoes, oregano, and red pepper flakes, and simmer uncovered until the mixture thickens slightly, about 30–40 minutes. If using canned lentils, add at this point, along with the basil. Cook an additional 3 minutes. Add salt and pepper to taste. Serve over wheel pasta; also good with vegetables, baked potatoes, beans, and grains.

LITE THOUSAND ISLAND DRESSING
Makes 1½ cups

1 10.5-oz package low-
  fat silken tofu
1 Tbs lemon juice
3 Tbs ketchup

2 Tbs sweet pickle relish
2 Tbs minced onion
1 tsp soy sauce

Place the tofu and lemon juice in a food processor or blender and process until smooth. Place in a bowl and stir in the remaining ingredients. Chill the dressing for about 2 hours before serving.

FRENCH BAKED POTATOES
—instead of greasy french fries!
Serves 2–4

3 medium potatoes
  (preferably organic)

1 Tbs olive oil in a
  spray bottle

Preheat the oven to 475 degrees. Use a nonstick flat baking pan, or line a pan with aluminum foil and spray lightly with oil. Wash and scrub the potatoes; don't peel. Cut each potato into ½-inch slices that are the full length of the potato. Place them on the sheet in a single layer. Spray potatoes lightly with oil. Bake 30–35 minutes until brown. Turn potatoes after 15 minutes. Sprinkle with salt, pepper, garlic salt, onion salt, or favorite herbs and serve.

30-MINUTE GUMBO

Serves 6

Make extra and freeze it in single serving–sized packages for
future meals.

1 large onion, chopped
4 cloves garlic, minced
1 green bell pepper,
chopped
2 stalks celery, sliced
6 cups vegetable broth
1 28-oz can Italian plum
tomatoes, chopped
(keep liquid)
2 tsp dried oregano
⅛ tsp cayenne pepper
1 10-oz package frozen
okra, chopped
1 10-oz package frozen
green beans

1 lb haddock fillets, cut
into 1-inch pieces, or
1 cup TSP (see "What
Is TSP?" on page
224)
1 cup frozen corn
2 cups cooked barley or
rice
¼ cup chopped fresh
parsley (optional
garnish)
Hot pepper sauce
(optional)

Place the onion, garlic, bell pepper, celery, and ½ cup
of the broth in a large saucepan and heat until soft-
ened, about 5 minutes. Add the remaining broth, tomatoes (and juice), oregano, and cayenne. Bring to a
boil. Reduce the heat and simmer for 5 minutes. Stir
in the okra and beans and simmer for 5 minutes. Raise
the heat until the mixture is boiling, add the fish, and
simmer 5 minutes; add corn. If not using fish, stir in
the corn and TSP together and heat through for 1–2

minutes; then turn off the heat, cover the pot, and let sit for 10 minutes before serving over the barley or rice. Parsley can be used as a garnish if desired.

WHAT IS TSP?

Textured soy protein (often referred to as TVP, texturized vegetable protein, a registered trademark of Archer Daniels Midland) is defatted soy flour that is made into dehydrated granules or chunks that you can rehydrate and add to recipes. Rehydrated TSP has a texture similar to ground beef (granules) or stew meat (chunks). TSP has little flavor of its own unless you buy flavored varieties, and absorbs the flavors of the ingredients in which it is cooked.

Don't think you've never eaten TSP. The ingredient lists of many foods include "textured soy flour" or "hydrolized vegetable protein," which is the same as TSP. It is high in protein, very low in fat and calories, and contains no cholesterol. One-half cup of prepared TSP, for example, contains about 24 grams of protein, only 0.2 gram of fat, and 160 calories. Three ounces of broiled ground beef contains about 245 calories, 18 grams of fat, and 20 grams of protein—plus cholesterol.

TSP is available in some supermarkets and most health food stores. Brand names include Archer Daniels Midland, Bob's Red Mill Natural Foods, So Soya, and Lumen Foods. You can also look on the Internet: www.soyfoods.com/cgi-bin/soyfoods.pl#3 and www.bulkfoods.com.

BREAKFAST MUFFINS

Makes 12 muffins

1 cup corn meal
1 cup whole wheat flour
2 tsp baking powder
¼ cup molasses or
  honey

1½ cups rice milk
2 Tbs applesauce
1 tsp egg replacer mixed
  with 2 Tbs water

In two separate bowls (one bowl should be large), combine the dry ingredients and the wet ingredients. Fold the dry and wet ingredients together and mix until moistened. Spoon the batter into nonstick muffin tins. Bake at 350 degrees for 30 minutes. Make a double batch and freeze the extras for quick breakfast treats.

STUFFED BAKED POTATOES

Serves 4

4 large baking potatoes,
  scrubbed
¼ cup vegetable broth
1 tsp olive oil
½ cup onion, finely
  chopped
2 cloves garlic, minced
¼ cup chopped red bell
  pepper

¼ cup chopped broccoli
½ cup mashed skim
  ricotta cheese or low-
  fat firm tofu
½ cup shredded low-fat
  cheese

Pierce the potatoes several times with a fork and place in a microwave on high for 15 to 20 minutes, turning once, until tender. While they are cooking, heat the broth and oil in a saucepan over medium heat. Add onion, garlic, bell pepper, and broccoli. Cook and stir often until vegetables begin to get soft, about 5 minutes. Remove from heat and stir in ricotta or tofu. Preheat broiler. Remove potatoes from the microwave and allow them to cool slightly. Place potatoes in a baking dish and split the tops open lengthwise. Spoon in the vegetable mixture and top each potato with cheese. Broil until the cheese melts, about 2 minutes.

WORLD'S FASTEST CHILI
Serves 4–6

3 15-oz cans of beans—
  kidney, pinto,
  black—your choice
  (keep juice)
1 cup of salsa, mild or
  moderate, depending
  on your taste

1 cup cooked lean
  ground turkey or
  TSP (see "What Is
  TSP?," page 224)
1 15-oz can corn (keep
  juice)

Place the beans (with juice), salsa, turkey or TSP, and corn (with juice) into a saucepan and bring to a boil; then reduce the heat and let simmer for 1–2 minutes. Add water if necessary. Turn off heat, cover pot, and let sit for 10 minutes.

GARLIC SALAD DRESSING

Makes 2 cups

*1 cup wine or cider
  vinegar*
1 cup water
2 Tbs lemon juice
2 cloves garlic
½ tsp celery seed

*1 small red onion, cut
  into chunks*
*1 small green pepper,
  seeded and cut into
  chunks*
½ tsp dill weed

Place all the ingredients into a blender and process until smooth. Refrigerate. This will keep several weeks in the refrigerator.

APPLE PIE

Serves 8

*One pie crust (see
  Blueberry Pie recipe,
  page 233)*
5 cups sliced apples
*⅓ cup thawed
  unsweetened apple
  juice concentrate*

1 tsp cinnamon
½ tsp nutmeg
½ cup flour
*½ cup thawed orange
  juice concentrate*
1 Tbs maple syrup
½ tsp baking powder

Prepare the pie crust according to instructions in the Blueberry Pie recipe. Leave the oven on 350 degrees, as you need to bake this pie.

    Place the apples, apple juice, cinnamon, and nutmeg in a saucepan. Bring to a boil and cook for about 5 minutes, stirring frequently. Remove from heat and pour into the pie crust. Combine the remaining ingredients in a separate bowl and sprinkle over the apples. Bake the pie for about 40 minutes.

BAKED BREADED FISH FILLETS
Seves 4

Skip the frozen, high-fat breaded fish fillets you'll find in your supermarket frozen food section and use this recipe instead.

2 cod or other fish fillets   4 Tbs dried seasoned
1 Tbs olive oil   bread crumbs

Preheat the oven to 400 degrees. Brush the fillets with the oil, then coat them with the crumbs. Place the fillets on a nonstick baking sheet. Bake until flaky, about 10 minutes. Instead of high-fat tartar sauce, serve with lemon juice or Lite Thousand Island Dressing (page 222).

ONION RINGS
Serves 2–4

Cooking oil spray, olive   ½ tsp each dried
    oil   oregano, cayenne
2 large onions   pepper, salt
¼ cup plain bread   ¼ tsp garlic powder
    crumbs   2 Tbs rice milk
2 Tbs corn meal

Preheat oven to 400 degrees. Lightly spray a flat baking sheet with the oil. Cut the onions into ½-inch thick slices. Separate the rings. In a bowl, combine the crumbs, corn meal, and seasonings. Dip each ring into the milk, then into the crumb mixture. Place on sheet. Bake 20 minutes, turning them after 10 minutes.

FRUIT SMOOTHIE
1 serving

*¼ cup applesauce,
  unsweetened*
1 tsp cinnamon

1 ripe banana
8 ounces of apple juice

Place all ingredients into a blender or food processor and blend until smooth.

MTM: MACARONI, TUNA, AND MUSHROOMS
Serves 4

This recipe is great left over for another night's dinner—or put extra into a thermos for lunch at work.

1 28-oz can tomatoes
2 cups water
*1½ cups dry pasta (your
  choice: elbows,
  bows, swirls)*
*1 6-oz can light tuna in
  water, drained*

*3 Tbs dried minced
  onion*
*1 cup fresh or canned
  mushrooms*
½ tsp salt
¼ tsp garlic powder

In a large saucepan, combine tomatoes and water and bring to a boil. Add the pasta, tuna, onion, mushrooms, salt, and garlic powder. Simmer, covered, for about 15 minutes or until the pasta is done. Stir occasionally, and add more water if necessary.

BROWNIES
Makes 16 brownies

1 cup unbleached flour	*1 cup Prune Puree (see*
²/₃ cup reduced fat cocoa	*recipe on page 239)*
powder or carob	*or Wonderslim Fat &*
powder	*Egg Replacer*
1 tsp baking powder	*1 cup sugar*
1 tsp baking soda	*1 tsp vanilla*
¼ tsp salt	*2 eggs*

Preheat oven to 350 degrees. Sift together the first five ingredients. In a separate bowl, combine the Prune Puree or Wonderslim and sugar. Stir in the vanilla. Whisk the eggs until frothy. Add to the sugar mixture and mix well. Add the wet ingredients to the dry ingredients and mix until blended. Spoon the mixture into a nonstick 8-inch baking dish and bake for 30 minutes.

BLACK AND WHITE SCRAMBLE
Serves 1

3 egg whites	*Soy sauce and pepper*
1 tsp olive oil	*to taste*
8 black olives, halved	

In a skillet, scramble the egg whites, olive oil, and olives until the eggs are firm. Season with soy sauce and pepper.

ANYTIME BISCUITS

Makes 8–10 biscuits

1 cup whole wheat flour
1½ tsp baking powder
½ tsp salt

⅓ cup nonfat milk
⅙ cup applesauce

Preheat oven to 450 degrees. Combine all the ingredients into a ball. Roll out on a floured board and cut with a biscuit cutter. Bake for about 8 minutes.

POTATO ENCHILADAS

Serves 4–6

2 16-oz cans or jars of
enchilada sauce
⅓ cup salsa
2 cups mashed potatoes
(instant is fine; use
water instead of milk;
no butter or oil)
8 whole wheat or soft
corn tortillas

¾ cup chopped green
onions
¾ cup corn kernels
(drain juice if you use
canned; or you can use
frozen corn, thawed)
1 4-oz can diced green
chilies

Preheat the oven to 350 degrees. Spread 1 cup of the enchilada sauce on the bottom of a casserole dish. Mix the salsa into the mashed potatoes. Spoon a line of the potatoes mixture down the center of each tortilla, then sprinkle with the onions, corn, and chilies. Roll up each tortilla and place seam side down in the casserole dish. Pour the remaining sauce over the tortillas, cover, and bake for 30 minutes.

POT PIE

Serves 4–6

2 extra large low-fat
flour tortillas
1 cup cubed chicken
breast (e.g., chicken
baked without oil, or
use canned chicken
breast in water, like
Swanson brand), or 1
cup mock chicken
strips (e.g., Lightlife
Chick 'n Strips)
2 Tbs soy sauce

2 Tbs water
1 cup finely chopped
onion
1 cup sliced celery
1 cup sliced carrots
1 cup any one of the
following: corn, peas,
mixed vegetables,
green beans,
zucchini, mushrooms
2 cups low-fat gravy
(recipe on next page)

Preheat the oven to 375 degrees. Place one of the tortillas in the bottom of an 8-inch pie plate and bake until the tortilla begins to harden, about 3–5 minutes. Remove from the oven. In a skillet, sauté the chicken in the soy sauce and water until lightly browned. Add the onion, celery, and carrots and continue to sauté until the onions are soft, about 5 minutes. Add the other vegetables and cook until all are tender, about 5 minutes.

Prepare the gravy (recipe follows). Pour it over the mixture in the skillet and stir. Pour the mixture into the pie pan and place the remaining tortilla on top of the mixture. Crimp the edges of the two tortillas together. Bake for 30 minutes or until the top tortilla is light brown.

LOW-FAT GRAVY

2 cups boiling water
2 Tbs olive or canola oil
(olive oil will give
gravy a different taste
than canola)
1 vegetable bouillon cube

½ cup diced fresh
mushrooms
½ cup finely chopped
onion
Flour

In a large saucepan, simmer all the ingredients except the flour for 5 minutes. Slowly add flour, one tablespoon at a time, and whisk until desired consistency is reached.

BLUEBERRY PIE

Serves 8

This recipe includes instructions to make the crust. Do not use commerically prepared pie crusts; they usually contain trans and saturated fats.

1½ cups Grape-Nuts
cereal (or a generic
equivalent that is fat
free)
1¼ cups thawed
unsweetened apple
juice concentrate
½ tsp vanilla
1 8-oz can unsweetened
crushed pineapple
(keep juice)

½ cup thawed
unsweetened grape
juice concentrate
¼ cup quick-cooking
tapioca
5 cups blueberries (fresh
or frozen)

Preheat the oven to 350 degrees. Make the crust by placing the cereal in a blender or food processor and processing it briefly until the kernels are slightly crushed. Combine ¾ cup apple juice concentrate with the vanilla. Place this mixture into a bowl and add the cereal. Mix well. Press the crust mixture into the bottom and sides of a 10-inch pie pan and bake for about 10–12 minutes. While the crust is baking, place the remaining apple juice, the pineapple and its juice, the grape juice, and the tapioca into a medium saucepan. Bring to a boil. Cook and stir until it becomes thick, about 3–4 minutes. Add the blueberries and cook for about 3 minutes. Pour the fruit mixture into the cooled crust and refrigerate the pie until it's thoroughly cooled.

CURRANTS AND CORNMEAL
Serves 4

4 cups water	*1 cup yellow cornmeal*
¾ cup currants	*½ cup chopped walnuts*
¼ tsp salt	*¼ cup raisins*

In a saucepan, bring water, currants, salt, and cornmeal to a boil, stirring frequently. When it reaches boiling, immediately lower the heat and simmer for 3–5 minutes. Stir often. Spoon into serving bowls and sprinkle with nuts and raisins.

VEGETABLE BEAN SOUP

Makes 8 servings

Make an extra batch; this soup freezes well.

2 potatoes
2 carrots
2 zucchini
1/4 lb green beans
8 cups of water
1 onion, chopped
2 cloves garlic, pressed
1/4 cup chopped parsley
1 tsp each basil and
   oregano

1/4 tsp each celery seed,
   marjoram, and pepper
1/4 lb red cabbage
1/3 cup brown rice
3 tomatoes, cut in
   quarters
1 can black beans (or
   kidney, pinto, navy)
Salt to taste

Scrub all the vegetables well (do not peel). Chop the potatoes into large chunks; slice carrots into 1/2-inch slices, zucchini into 1-inch slices, and green beans into 1-inch pieces. Place into a large pot; add the water. Also add the chopped onion, garlic, and seasonings (except salt). Simmer for one hour. Add the thinly sliced cabbage and rice. Simmer for 20–25 minutes, then add the tomato pieces and the canned beans. Add more water if the soup is too thick. Add salt to taste. Simmer for an additional 10 minutes and serve.

WHOLE WHEAT CRACKERS

Makes about 48 crackers

½ cup whole wheat flour
2 Tbs applesauce
2 Tbs sunflower seeds

⅛ tsp salt
½ cup cottage cheese

Preheat the oven to 350 degrees. Combine all the ingredients except the cottage cheese in a blender and process until fine crumbs. Place the crumbs into a bowl. Process the cottage cheese until smooth. Return the crumbs to the blender and process with the cottage cheese until a ball forms. Roll out the dough on a floured board until it is even and about ¼-inch thick. Prick the dough all over with a fork. Cut the dough crosswise into four equal strips, then lengthwise into three equal strips, then into fourths, for a total of about 48 crackers. Bake for 20 mintues.

PIZZA

Serves 1

Forget the high-fat pizzas from the supermarket or the pizzeria around the corner. Stay at home and make this quick and easy pizza in minutes.

1 large whole wheat
* tortilla*
½ cup marinara sauce
Choice of toppings: sliced
* black olives, sautéed*
* green peppers and*
* onions, sautéed*
* mushrooms*

Garlic powder and dried
* oregano (optional)*
½ cup shredded low-fat
* cheese*

Preheat oven to 450 degrees. Place the tortilla on a nonstick pizza pan. Spread the sauce on the tortilla, add your favorite toppings, sprinkle with garlic powder and/or dried oregano to taste, and then sprinkle with the cheese. Bake until the cheese melts, about 5 minutes.

SNACK RECIPES

NO BAKE CRISPY BARS
Makes about 25 bars

4 cups breakfast cereal that has flakes and dried fruit, such as Kellogg's Fruit Harvest or Kashi Organic Promise
1 Tbs ground flaxseed

½ cup chopped walnuts
1 cup chunky peanut butter, preferably natural
½ cup brown rice syrup
3 Tbs brown sugar

In a large bowl, combine cereal, flaxseed and chopped walnuts. In a saucepan, combine peanut butter, syrup, and brown sugar. Stir over medium heat until creamy. Pour over the cereal mixture and stir until the cereal is evenly covered. Spoon the mixture into a lightly oiled 8x8 inch baking pan and press down firmly. Allow the mixture to cool for about 15 mintues, then cut into squares.

CHOCOLATE PUDDING

Serves 6–8

2 10.5-oz packages of
low-fat silken tofu
(Mori-Nu Silken Lite
Extra Firm is
suggested)
½ cup low-fat cocoa
powder

¾ cup honey or maple
syrup (maple syrup
will give the pudding a
different taste than
will the honey)
3 tsp vanilla

Place the tofu into a food processor and process until
smooth. Place the cocoa powder into a bowl. Microwave the honey or maple syrup until it is liquidy,
about 1 minute. Pour this liquid over the cocoa and
mix together until smooth. Add this mixture and the
vanilla to the blended tofu in the food processor and
process again until very smooth. Pour into serving
dishes and refrigerate for at least 4 hours.

TRANS FAT–FREE BAKING SUBSTITUTE: FRUIT!

You can eliminate the use of shortening, butter,
and margarine when baking by using fat-free fruit
baking substitutes. The easiest one to use is unsweetened applesauce, which is inexpensive, readily
available, and has very little effect on the final flavor of whatever you add it to. Because applesauce
contains more pectin than other fruit substitutes, it

helps your baked goods stay moist. Pectin is a naturally occurring substance in fruit; it acts similar to solid shortening that has been added to a recipe that contains sugar.

Besides applesauce, you can also use other fruits, including mashed ripe bananas, mashed cooked pumpkin, and pureed prunes (recipe below). You can also mix and match any of these fruits in a recipe.

The important thing to remember about substituting fruits for shortening in a recipe is to use one half of the amount the original recipe calls for. For example, if a muffin recipe calls for ½ cup margarine, use ¼ cup of applesauce or other mashed fruit or puree.

Here's the recipe for prune puree:

1 12-oz package pitted prunes
¼ cup light corn syrup
¾ cup water

Place the prunes and corn syrup in a food processor and process slightly. Slowly add the water while processing and continue to process and add the water until you have a smooth consistency. Store the puree in a covered container in the refrigerator.

Appendix

Would you like to know more about the food you're eating? You can contact the consumer service department of food manufacturers and fast-food restaurants and request nutritional information. Contact information for individual food items from the supermarket can usually be found on the packaging. Many provide a phone number and/or Web site; some provide an address only. If you wish to contact a fast-food restaurant, you can ask for the consumer service department phone number from a store manager, or access the information on the Internet. To help you get started, we have researched various food manufacturers and fast-food restaurants and listed their contact information below.

FOOD MANUFACTURERS

Aurora Foods, Inc., makers of Aunt Jemima, Celeste, Duncan Hines, Lender's, Mrs. Paul's, Van de Kamp's, and other brands.

- For Aunt Jemima, Celeste, Lender's, and Mrs. Paul's, write to Aurora Foods, 11432 Lackland Road, St. Louis MO 63146.
- For Duncan Hines, call 1-800-845-7286.
- For Van de Kamp's, write to Consumer Affairs, PO Box 66884, St. Louis MO 63166.

Campbell's Soup Company, makers of Campbell's soups, Franco-American foods, Pepperidge Farm products, V-8, Swanson broths, Prego, and other brands 1-800-257-8443

Fantastic Foods
1-800-288-1089

Green Giant
1-800-998-9996

Healthy Choice (a ConAgra Foods brand)
1-800-323-9980

Kashi
1-858-274-8870

Kellogg's
1-800-962-1413

Kraft Foods, makers of Athenos, Chips Ahoy!, Cream of Wheat, General Foods International Coffees, Honey Maid, Kraft salad dressings, Kraft Macaroni & Cheese, Lunchables, Oscar Mayer, Oreo,

Philadelphia Cream Cheese, Planters nuts, Post cereals, Ritz crackers, Tombstone pizzas, Velveeta, among other brands 1-800-323-0768

Nestlé
Hand-Held Food Groups (Hot Pockets, Lean Pockets, Croissant Pockets, Pot Pie Express)
1-800-350-5016

Newman's Own
246 Post Road East
Westport, CT 06880

Pillsbury
1-800-775-4777

Quaker Oats Co.
1-800-234-6281 (cold cereals)
1-800-555-6287 (Instant Quaker Oats)

Stouffers
1-800-225-1180
Stouffer's Lean Cuisine: 1-800-993-8625

Swanson
1-800-768-6287

Uncle Ben's
1-800-548-6253

Unilever Best Foods

- For Breyers and Good Humor, contact www.icecreamusa.com
- For Brummel & Brown, I Can't Believe It's Not Butter, Imperial Spread, and Shedd's Spread, call 1-800-735-3554
- For Hellmann's, Skippy, Knorr, call 1-800-338-8831
- For Lipton and Wish-Bone, call 1-800-697-7887
- For Ragú, call 1-800-328-7748
- For Slim-Fast, contact www.slim-fast.com

FAST-FOOD RESTAURANTS

Arby's
1-800-487-2729

Boston Market
1-800-365-7000

Burger King
1-305-378-3535
www.burgerking.com

Dairy Queen
1-952-830-0200
www.dairyqueen.com

Jack in the Box
1-800-955-5225
www.jackinthebox.com

KFC
1-800-225-5532
www.kfc.com

Pizza Hut
1-800-948-8488
www.pizzahut.com

Subway
1-800-888-4848
www.subway.com

Taco Bell
1-800-822-6235
www.tacobell.com

Wendy's
1-614-764-3100
www.wendys.com

OTHER RESTAURANT/FOOD CHAINS

Applebee's
1-888-592-7753
www.applebees.com

Appendix

Big Boy
1-800-837-3003
www.bigboy.com

Carrows
1-877-225-4161
www.carrows.com

Chi-Chi's
1-800-436-6006
www.chi-chis.com

Cracker Barrel
1-615-444-5533
www.crackerbarrel.com

Denny's
1-800-733-6697
www.dennys.com

Dunkin' Donuts
1-877-833-2633
www.dunkindonuts.com

Houlihan's
1-816-756-2200
www.houlihans.com

IHOP
1-818-240-6055
www.ihop.com

Marie Callender's
1-800-776-7437
www.mcpies.com

The Olive Garden
1-800-331-2729
www.theolivegarden.com

Panda Express
1-800-877-8988
www.pandaexpress.com

Red Lobster
1-800-562-7837
www.redlobster.com

Starbucks
1-206-447-1575
www.starbucks.com

T.G.I. Friday's
1-800-374-3297
www.tgifridays.com

Village Inn
1-303-296-2121
www.yourvillageinn.com

Deborah Mitchell is a medical writer and journalist whose articles have appeared in professional journals as well as national consumer magazines. She has authored or coauthored two dozen books dealing with topics in health and nutrition. Ms. Mitchell is an experienced collaborator, a meticulous researcher, and is highly skilled at making complex technical information easy to understand. She lives with her husband, four cats, and three dogs in the desert outside of Tucson, Arizona.